DATE DUE

SEP 1 9 2001	
JUL 1 7 2003	
AUG 1 0 2003	
AUG 2 8 2003	
9/21/03	
DEC 1 8 2003	
FEB 1 0 2004	
AUG 1 8 2006	

DEMCO, INC. 38-2931

THE *New*

BEVERLY HILLS DIET

The latest weight-loss research that explains
a conscious food-combining program for
LIFELONG SLIMHOOD

JUDY MAZEL

and Michael Wyatt
with medical commentary by Albert Sokol, M.D.

Health Communications, Inc.
Deerfield Beach, Florida

The New Beverly Hills Diet is not intended as a substitute for the medical advice of physicians. The reader should regularly consult a physician in matters relating to his or her health and especially, with respect to any symptoms that may require diagnosis. Any eating regimen, including this one, should be undertaken only under the direct supervision of the reader's physician. In particular, this regimen should not be followed by anyone who has certain diseases or conditions, including, without limitation, diabetes, colitis, hypoglycemia, a spastic colon, ulcers, ileitis, enteritis, diverticulosis or by anyone who is pregnant or breast feeding. Moreover, anyone with other chronic or serious ailments or who is under treatment for a medical condition, should undertake this eating program only under the direct supervision of his or her own physician.

Library of Congress Cataloging-in-Publication Data

Mazel, Judy.
The new Beverly Hills diet/Judy Mazel.
 p. cm.
ISBN 1-55874-425-8 (trade paper).—ISBN 1-55874-431-2 (hbk.)
1. Reducing diets. 2. Food combining. I. Title
RM222.2.M42   1996   96-33480
613.'5—dc20   CIP

Publisher: Health Communications, Inc.
          3201 S.W. 15th Street
          Deerfield Beach, FL 33442-8190

Cover design by Lawna Patterson Oldfield

For my mother
with the hope that her 80th birthday wish
comes true

Contents

Acknowledgments

My words cannot express
How much you share in the success
The love and gratitude that fill my heart
Recalling how you played a part

Thank you . . .

Bikram Choudhury for strength of commitment, an understanding of waves and an inpenetrable bullet-proof vest

Cintra Brown for sending me straight to the source

Margie and Herman Platt for your unconditional love

Rick Goldstein for being in the right place at the right time wearing very shiny armour

Patti Rose and Esther Reifer for forts in the storm

Peter Vegso for a terrific birthday

Mike Wyatt for having a genius weigh with words and Holly

Leslie Dillihunt and Lightening for everything

Carol Maizel for your CONFIDENCE

Gene Rosenbaum for missing the boat and setting my course

David Eddy for being there

Don Flynn and Michele Raffner XTEL Communications for keeping the lines open

Remy Smith for her one room with a futon

Frances Wymore for saving the day(s)

Jodi Nusser for fonts, anchors and keeping my arrows straight

Carla Becker for loving buffets

Matthew Diener for drums of steel

Kim Weiss and Kim Morgan for spreading the word

Jerry Criscuolo for a pot of gold at the end of the rainbow and Rosa Mezistrano for sunny skies

Don Allen and Lori Helton for champion ribs; Steve Messerer and Kristie Laufer—Erica Robertson and Micki Paul for nuts and bolts/copies and cash; Ana Lisa Bautista and Julie Martin for care, feeding and feedback; and Judy Deignan for "sweet" smiles

Jennifer Jordan & Emily Lenzner for taking a nibble; Cary Butler for a big bite; and Lynette Nutter for reeling it in

Heath Carnes, Dan Tomlinson, Bob Bour, Ray Russo and Hugh Devlin for YOU, your very special Inn at Queen Anne, and my Samadhi

Rabbi Allan Shrantz for planting the seed

Janie Greenspun Gail for starting it all

and

Guruji Paramahansa Yogananda, for getting me to the shore without drowning

Next book, I hope I'll have you to thank for being my best example . . .

SKINNY doesn't mean sticks and bones.

SKINNY is when you can get on the scale and you don't have to say, "If only . . ." "If only I could lose 10 pounds" or "I'd be perfect if . . ." "I'd be perfect if I could lose a few pounds."

SKINNY means perfect in your own eyes. Whatever your weight is!

Preface

An estimated 60 million Americans are overweight. It is safe to say that most of them are not happy about it. They have:

- tried fad diets time and time again
- pummeled their bodies in gyms and health clubs
- deprived themselves of the food they love
- followed rigid programs of self-denial and sacrifice in pursuit of a promised result that has proved elusive

And nothing has worked. Despite their best efforts and their most fervent hopes, nothing has worked to give them the body they want—and let them keep it. Until now.

The weight is over!

Introduction

It has been 15 years since the publication of my original *The Beverly Hills Diet*. Never in my wildest dreams did I ever think I would be writing *The New Beverly Hills Diet*.

Millions of people lost weight while on my original diet. They learned about Conscious Combining, the foundation of my diet, and developed a healthy eating lifestyle that has kept them thin. I, too, have learned. Through 15 years of refining, fine-tuning and broadening my technique of Conscious Combining, I have learned just how expansive it can be.

What's new about *The New Beverly Hills Diet?*

The original *The Beverly Hills Diet* was a book that was read in one or two sittings and was referred back to as a guide.

The New Beverly Hills Diet is a day-to-day support system, a hand-holding guide you interact with each day.

The New Beverly Hills Diet is not a diet; it's a lifestyle eating plan, a plan that focuses on the individual adoption of the technique of Conscious Combining, the technique I first introduced in *The Beverly Hills Diet* in 1981.

The New Beverly Hills Diet represents 15 years of research and experimentation; keeping a close eye on the progress of clients; taking copious notes; refining, modifying, fine-tuning, expanding and stretching the original premise of Conscious Combining to its fullest potential.

The original *The Beverly Hills Diet* began with 10 days of fruit and did not include animal protein until day 19. *The New Beverly Hills Diet* includes foods from all food groups in the first week, including animal protein, meeting all standards set by the U.S. Senate Committee on Nutrition and Human Needs as recommended for a balanced weekly diet.

In the first week of *The New Beverly Hills Diet* you will eat corn on the cob, baked potatoes (butter included), pasta, fresh fruit, steak, shrimp (or animal protein of choice), salads with real oil and vinegar salad dressing. There is no portion control, and you can even have wine and champagne if desired.

My original *The Beverly Hills Diet* was a structured 42-day eating regimen that allowed for very limited eating deviations or choices. *The New Beverly Hills Diet* encourages open eating with guidance. There are 21 open-choice meals in the 35-day regimen

My original *The Beverly Hills Diet* had only 9 protein meals in 42 days. On *The New Beverly Hills Diet* you can double that to 18, depending on the choices *you* make.

My recent innovations, however, are not my only reasons for writing this new book. Unfortunately, over the past decade food processing and preparation have become hazards to our health. Artificial coloring, the rampant use of hydrogenated and partially hydrogenated oils (cottonseed and/or palm kernel), artificial flavorings, growth hormones (legal and illegal), preservatives, high salt levels, imitation fats and fast foods, just to name a few, have become a part of the daily diets of too many Americans.

Not the least of these problems is an epidemic of obesity. Obesity not only touches our adult population, but affects our children as well, including babies fed formulas lacking real nutritional substance, and containing hydrogenated and partially hydrogenated oil as well. Our increasingly busy lifestyles have caused us to let down our guard. We, as a society, have given free license to big business, in the name of convenience and taste, to do as they please with our food supply.

The figures are shocking. Eighty percent of Americans are overweight. Obviously "fad" diets, calorie counting, medically sanctioned, prescribed pills and powders do not work. Statistics show that 98 percent of all dieters gain back their lost pounds, plus more, within a year!

The alarm must go out. Obesity is at the very forefront of our nation's health crisis. It not only costs millions of Americans their health and happiness, but medical problems related to obesity annually run up millions of dollars in health care costs. And this crisis not only afflicts America, where one in three adults over the age of 30 and one in five children are classified as clinically obese: its effects are felt across the rest of the industrialized world as well. This is a global problem.

My book and its message are an answer. Definitely not a "diet," as we have come to think of diets, my program offers instead an opportunity to take charge of the food you eat and to effectively combine these foods for optimum nutrition and slimhood. Within this book is a lifestyle eating plan that will not only turn you into a Born-Again Skinny, but will give you healthy eating habits to keep you that way forever.

The New Beverly Hills Diet, however, is not just about learning how to combine foods. It is also about nutrition, food selection, food preparation and exercise. It is a simple 35-day eating program that is comprised of "real" food and "real" nutritional information. My 35-day weight-loss program not only gets you thin, it provides you with a launching pad to a healthier life. It is the foundation for the development and maintenance of an eating lifestyle that will keep you slim forever.

The New Beverly Hills Diet is a wake-up call that will turn you into a Born-Again Skinny forever!

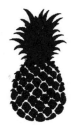

PART I

Welcome to Lifelong Slimhood

The Weight Is Over

Hamburgers and hipbones. . . . Cheesecake and cheekbones. . . . There's a pot of gold at the end of the rainbow called Eternal Slimhood: a land where you can be as thin as you'd like for the rest of your life.

Welcome to the world of dreams come true—to a "diet" that's a dream come true. This is *The New Beverly Hills Diet* lifestyle eating program. This is a program with no portion control and no forbidden foods, a program that actually allows you to indulge yourself and your every food fantasy. Hot dogs at the ball game, French fries and a shake. At last you can go public and have that affair out in the open . . . with food. Believe me, I know about food. I, too, love to eat, and I live to eat. When food is in my mouth, my heart sings and my soul soars. I can match you food fantasy for food fantasy, bite for bite. I'm no different than you. Well, maybe a little bit, because I'm thin now. But you will be, too, once I've taught you how.

Can you imagine yourself in a world where you don't have to count calories or measure portions? A world with no "no's," no "never's," no forbidden foods. A world where you don't have to cheat to eat anything, even if that anything is a chocolate-chip cheesecake. Welcome to the world of Born-Again Skinny.

Try to imagine yourself being as thin as you have ever wanted to be, eating the way you want to eat, standing at the sink, driving in your car, even at the refrigerator with the door open! Oh no, I'm not going to limit you to three meals a day with no snacks in between. You won't have to eat off smaller plates, leave half your food or put your fork down between bites. You won't have to modify your behavior, and you don't have to go through psychoanalysis to understand why you eat. The "why" isn't important. It doesn't matter. What is important is that you'll never go hungry, nor will you have to give up your favorite foods to have the body you've always longed for, the body that will soon be yours—if you are willing to give up three things: (1) your guilt; (2) your fat; and (3) all of your preconceived ideas, everything you've ever been taught to believe about fat and fattening, diets and dieting, because being thin has nothing to do with what you eat, or how much you eat, but rather when you eat and what foods you eat together.

For the next 35 days you'll experience a way of eating that I first developed for myself, my way of going from 180 pounds to my current 108. It is a way of eating I have taught to millions of readers and hundreds of personal clients—Liza Minelli, Jack Nicholson, Jodie Foster and Maria Shriver, to mention a few. You are going to learn that nothing has to be fattening, not even a piece of pepperoni pizza with extra cheese. You see, it's all in the enzymes.

Let me explain. The human body is activated by enzymes, biological catalysts that appear in the food you eat or are promoted in your body by the food you eat. There are three food groups: (1) proteins; (2) carbohydrates; and (3) fats. Each has its own set of enzymes. A protein enzyme works on proteins, a carbohydrate enzyme works on carbohydrates, and a fat enzyme works on fats. Not only can they not cross over (a protein enzyme can't work on a carbohydrate, a carbohydrate enzyme can't work on a protein), but the presence of one can destroy the effect of the other.

So what does this have to do with your weight? Enzymes break down food so that your body can properly and efficiently digest it. I base my whole technique for eating on the thesis that when food is not properly digested, it turns into excess weight. When you mix too many foods from the different food groups together (the proteins, the carbohydrates, the fats)—your basic balanced meal—you confuse the enzymes and this prompts a weight gain.

This is just a thumbnail sketch. We will go into much more detail as we go along.

On *The New Beverly Hills Diet* you'll learn to make your enzymes work for you by eating foods together that should go together and counteracting those that don't. This includes all the foods you've been eating and would like to continue eating. You know, all those "fattening" foods. However, the difference will be that you will eat them in certain specific combinations and you'll see how the right combination of foods can trigger astonishing weight loss and weight maintenance. Some of the foods you will be eating may seem foreign to you at first, such as the papayas and mangoes, and some I'm sure will be foods you never thought you'd be able to eat on a weight-loss program (pastas, corn on the cob and baked potatoes with butter, avocados and even desserts).

If you just do what I say and eat what I tell you to eat (believe me, I won't let you go hungry), you'll soon see that a thin, healthy world exists beyond the skinless chicken breast, the dry broiled fish and that ever-familiar "diet plate." Because this is unlike any diet you've ever been on, this is the last diet you will ever go on. This time you'll get thin and you'll stay thin, no bones about it! Unless, of course, it's those hipbones that are going to emerge from under those mountains of flesh. I'm going to teach you a way of eating that's going to change your life, just as it changed mine and oh-so-many others.

Never again will you have to go to bed hungry, feeling deprived, deprived of all the foods you love or the body you long to have. You can have both—hamburgers and hipbones, cheesecake and cheekbones—all the foods you love and the body you've always dreamed of. In the next five weeks, you are going to eat food, all kinds of food, even the most fattening food. That includes all your favorites, all of those foods that you've always had to break a diet to eat. You'll see that when those foods are properly combined with other foods, not only will you not gain weight, you'll lose weight.

Your initial weight loss is going to be achieved by eating very specific foods in a very specific order.

Although most of your meals will be scheduled for the next 35 days, you'll have 21 opportunities to "go for it," to eat the foods you love, no matter what they happen to be—fried chicken and mashed potatoes, even apple pie à la mode—and you'll see how you'll lose weight by feeding your body, not by starving it, and how you'll maintain that weight loss the same way. It is food that's going to get you thin and keep you thin . . . not pills, not some chemical powder in a can or prepackaged meals. Just food, glorious food. Life, my soon-to-be-skinny friend, is like a smorgasbord; a world of taste treats and eating experiences. A bite here, a nibble there, sit down for a meal, stop for a snack. Your choices are wide open and the sky's the limit! And, believe me, there is pie in the sky, and you can have your cake and eat it too. Food and eating and the body you've always longed to have are yours for the taking.

It doesn't matter if you travel, go out to dinner every night, have business lunches, love Sunday brunches, eat when you are stressed, depressed, high or low. None of these things will stop you from being the thinnest you've ever wanted to be, not once you've adopted and adapted my exciting and unique way of eating. And as you do, you'll see that the excuses, along with the pounds, will disappear.

It doesn't matter who you are, where you live, what your life is like or how much money you have in the bank. If you are willing to accept that whatever you've been doing, on or off your diet, just isn't working, that you still aren't the weight you want to be no matter how hard you've tried; and if you accept that there is another way, and believe in it, then I promise you, if you just give me 35 days of your life and commit to following my program to the letter, you will not fail! You'll get thin and you'll stay thin, once and for all and forever.

Oh, by the way, from now on you have a new name. You don't mind if I call you Skinny, do you?

Life in the Slim Lane

Hello, Skinny, or soon to be. You are on your way with *The New Beverly Hills Diet* program. No, you are not going on another diet. You are embarking on a lifestyle eating program, a program that's going to take you off the fat track so you can start living life in the slim lane.

As you already know, lifelong lifestyle changes, particularly eating changes, aren't easy, and they don't happen just by simply reading about them. They happen one day at a time, and they happen by doing them. This is precisely how you'll proceed with your new lifestyle eating program and reading the second half of my book—one day at a time.

You'll find that the first part of this book follows a traditional format. It is divided into chapters, each with its own heading and subject. These chapters provide you with all the facts and figures, the "why's" and the "wherefore's." They contain all the intellectual ammunition you'll need to fight the Battle of the

Bulge! A battle from which you'll finally emerge victorious because I will be there with you each step of the way.

Rejoice! Fat will cease to be your enemy and, at long last, food will truly become your best friend.

In the second part of the book, "Born-Again Skinny," we will really get down to the nitty-gritty; the *bare bones.* Call it your daily bread . . . a nibble at night before you go to sleep; a big bite in the morning when you wake up; our own one-on-one sessions, not unlike the short daily chats I have with my private clients. These chapters will only take you about 10 minutes to read. However, it is in those 10 minutes that we spend together that you'll learn to apply my techniques, as well as receive all the intellectual and emotional support you'll need to get through the day. Not that it's going to be particularly difficult. What's so difficult about eating baked potatoes and corn on the cob dripping in butter? Who would object to dining on a pasta dinner with no portion control, steaks as big as you please, shrimp cocktails with sauce, or salads as large as you desire with as much oil as you want? This is hardly what you'd describe as hard time in diet prison. And that's just the first week.

You'll see, it will be just as I promised you. You won't go hungry! Believe me, I won't ever let you leave the table feeling deprived, feeling that you haven't had enough or that you are a terrible person because you still want more. Eat away! No matter how big your appetite, you'll *still* get thin and, more important, you will stay thin.

Never again will you have to worry about the size of your portions, cut the fat off your steak, skin your chicken or even consider giving up the foods you love so much. All those foods will be a part of these next 35 days.

Imagine what it will be like to look forward to getting on the scale. Imagine what it will be like to look at yourself in the mirror and see the body you have always fantasized having. Imagine never being fat again—ever!

Well, get ready for an adventure: an adventure into the world of food, eating and feeling good. Feeling good physically, spiritually and emotionally can be yours by confronting, acknowledging and letting go of your fat person and letting your Skinny soul soar. By developing a Skinny voice that's going to out-shout the screaming, strident voice of fat.

Trust me, rely on me and, most important, trust your "Skinny" self. I promise you, if you read my book the way it was intended to be read, the way I tell you to read it, and follow my instructions, you will not fail. You will internalize it, you will synthesize it, and all your dreams will come true. THIN will at long last be a forever reality.

It is the enthusiasm of my new Born-Again Skinnies that nourishes my program, reinforces its validity and propels me to devote my life to its perpetuation and the abolition of the fat consciousness that pervades so many of us. Here's what some of them have to say about the program:

I've been trying to lose weight and keep it off for 20 years. I've gone from a size 18 to a size 14, and I'm so sure I will never gain it back again, I've thrown out all my old clothes.

—Ramonia F., Maryland

Before I started your diet I was 197 pounds and only 5' ½" tall. I'm still 5' ½" tall, but now I weigh 160 pounds. I've lost 37 pounds. My goal is to lose a total of 82 pounds. I only have 45 more to go, and this will be a piece of cake. I'm sharing this diet with others so that they may feel good about themselves, as I do. Thank you, Judy.

—Barbara R., New York

Losing weight, positive body consciousness and feeling good about oneself are not limited to women; men have these same feelings, too.

I'm writing to tell you how successful your new diet is. It is a long road, but it is not the long road I thought it would be . . . I've lost 16 pounds so far. Thank you for making me look and feel better.

—Matt S., Florida

I'm a recently divorced and retired business executive whose current lifestyle allows the focus to be on what's really important . . . myself. I discovered your New Beverly Hills Diet and thought I would give it a try. Obtaining the foods you designated presented no problem even for a neophyte shopper like myself. In six weeks I lost 26 pounds. Please allow me to say thank you, and to spread your gospel.

—Bob F., Ohio

I've been on the diet for two weeks and lost nine pounds without being hungry. I feel great, I look great, and I will recommend this diet to anyone. P.S. After two weeks of fine dining with friends and family in Europe, I still haven't gained back a pound.

—Stephan A., Florida

If you agree never to starve yourself and stop thinking of potatoes and pasta as fattening; if lobster and butter are more exciting than chicken without the skin; if corn on the cob and avocados have more appeal than cottage cheese and tomato slices; if popcorn sounds like more fun than carrot sticks, then *The New Beverly Hills Diet* will work for you too.

The New Beverly Hills Diet *has enabled me to lose 26 pounds in 43 days, despite a week of indiscretion when I was rebelling against fruit or something. I have never lost weight this easily before. I look forward to trying to maintain this combining system because I do love an occasional piece of cheesecake or pasta with olive oil and garlic. I would rather eat a lot of fruit and be able to use real oil, butter and sour cream than eat limited portions of diet foods and oil imitations. Granted, some of the days are boring, but what diet isn't? I would certainly rather have an avocado and tomato sandwich with a good spread of mayo than a one-ounce meat and veggie sandwich on diet bread with my allowed teaspoon of fat or a poached egg any day. My brothers keep saying how great I look. Wait until they see me at my annual Fourth of July party; I will make that a protein day and eat all the ribs and chicken I want.*

—Lisa S., Maine

I've been trying to lose about 20 pounds for six months. I tried stopping the insanity to no avail. I heard about The New Beverly Hills Diet, where I could eat real food and lose weight. I tried it and was amazed at the results; 9 pounds the first week and 3 pounds each week thereafter for a total of 20 pounds. I ate a variety of foods, from duck pizza to veal romana with pasta; chicken parmigiana; a corned beef, pastrami, chopped liver platter with rye bread and potato pancakes; steak and lobster with real butter. I even drank beer and vodka as well as champagne and, of course, I ate a lot of fruit. I will continue to follow the diet to lose an additional six to eight pounds and then go on maintenance. Since I started, quite a few people have joined me and have had great results. My daughter, Samantha, lost 12 pounds in three weeks. I would recommend this plan for anyone wishing to lose weight while eating everyday food.

—Marty B., Florida

You'll learn that "blowing it" is a thing of the past. You don't have to eat yourself under the table anymore because there is nothing on that table that you can't have. The trick is learning how and when to eat, and what to do to compensate for it.

I was delighted to learn that The New Beverly Hills Diet *was not really a diet but a way of combining foods to enhance the digestive process. After five weeks I was two dress sizes smaller and happy as a clam because I can eat this way forever and be forever thin.*

—Anne A., Florida

You cannot blow it because Judy teaches you how to consciously combine your meals. You properly combine foods and then use the corrective counterpart. It is actually fun. You must, however, have a plan. You plan to eat what you want, how and when. It all hinges on three little words: how, when, what.

—Marian S., Mexico

You'll learn to make every bite count, to experience food and make it an experience, to think about food when it doesn't count, so you don't have to think about it when it does.

I've learned a whole new way of eating. I've learned to eat fruit that I never thought I'd eat. I've learned to think before I put just anything into my mouth. I've learned to like myself again. I look at people, watching them eat, and think to myself, "If you only knew."

—Dee G., Florida

You'll understand and appreciate that food, wonderful restaurants and everything about eating will be here tomorrow. If you don't have it now, you can have it later; if not later, tomorrow.

My life is one big round of cocktail parties, luncheons and charity balls. All those delectable party foods had settled in a 15-pound ring around my middle. Then, I tried your diet. Now 12 pounds lighter, I feel great, know a lot about nutrition, have stopped eating things just because I'm there and so are they, and I've quit looking for the book that promises to change my life. Yours did, and I love it. Just keep calling me Skinny.
—Barbara M., Florida

Although I'm not at my goal yet, I'm sure I will be shortly and, more important, I will be able to maintain it. I feel good being thinner, I look good being thinner and, most of all, I'm in control, something that has not been true for me for years. Although I completely agree with your program, that doesn't mean I've resolved all my diet problems. I just don't have to go crazy now when I have a bad day. Just because there's a blizzard, I don't have to eat everything in sight. I now know that "nothing is leaving the planet," and I can have anything I want if I plan for it.
—Rae, New York

How many pounds have you lost in your life and then regained? Aren't you ready to lose them now, once and for all, forever? Well, they did it, they got thin. I did it, and I got thin. So will you!

THREE

Fat to Fabulous

For the last 19 years, my five-foot, four-inch frame hasn't wavered more than a few pounds from its ideal weight of 108 pounds. But I haven't always been the thin, svelte person that I am today. . . . I was once 180 pounds of a bloated, beached whale. Actually, I'm exaggerating. The true figure is $177^3/_4$. However, just saying that number still makes me shudder at the recollection of the day I was confronted with it.

I can still see the doctor's face as he stood back from the scale, arms folded across his chest, nostrils flaring as his eyes filled with thinly veiled revulsion. "One hundred seventy-seven and three-quarters," he stated in a flat, nasal tone. My fat, naked body blushed bright red in humiliation at his gaze.

I wanted to die! It wasn't just a number; it was a judgment. I never went to another diet doctor again. He was the last in a chain of many; the end of 20 years of agony as a fatty and the birth of a Born-Again Skinny.

You see, I wasn't born fat; I just got that way. I became a fat child in a family of skinnies, at a time when fat children were a minority. In fact, there were only two in my class . . . and I was one of them.

I was taken to my first "diet doctor" at the age of nine, and for the next 20 years I was on a roller-coaster ride of wild ups and downs. Taking a diet pill each morning was as normal as brushing my teeth. Unfortunately, back in the 1950s, doctors were prescribing amphetamines and were somewhat indiscriminate about doling out thyroid medication to speed up "slow metabolisms."

Not only did the medication not make me thin, it did little to enhance my personality or my sleep habits. Unknowingly wired with "speed," I'd report my inability to sleep to my mother. She would suggest counting sheep. "But Mom, I can't count that high," I'd reply. I was nervous and moody. The medication made my head ache, and my weight made my heart ache. I was considered high-strung and difficult, a real brat! No one even considered or realized that it was the massive doses of amphetamines that were convoluting my personality.

As a child I bounced between fat and chubby as I picked my way through a merry-go-round of diet doctors, shots, pills, diets, diets and more diets. Everybody watched what I ate. And, in turn, what I ate increasingly dominated my life. My home life was a menu of mixed messages. Food, love, fat and family were all mixed up. Meanwhile, I loved to clear the table because that was my chance to grab everybody's leftovers. My family constantly nagged. "Are you still eating, Judy?" "Haven't you had enough,

Judy?" The more they nagged, the more I ate.

My teen and young adult years were just more of the same. Oh, I'd have brief moments of slimhood only to get fat all over again. Back I'd go to yet another diet doctor, sitting in the quiet office with a line of other fatties, all of us looking for the cure.

Along with each new doctor and diet came newer and "more effective" weight control medications. With dieting, my focus on food only increased. I'd steal bits of change from my mother's purse during the week so that I'd have money for pizza when I was left alone on my dateless Saturday nights. Those evenings alone began with the intense pleasure of food and ended with the intensely painful guilt of hidden food wrappers and the knowledge that I had somehow betrayed the trust of my family.

As I entered adulthood, the pills kept me controlled at somewhere between 140 and 165 pounds. My weight fluctuated depending on the day of the week, my emotional life and my social calendar. Every Monday I'd start a diet. Sometimes I'd even make it to Friday . . . but weekends were another story.

Friday night would begin with a vodka martini with two—no, make it three—olives and a twist. Then it was an à la carte meal of anything that wasn't nailed down. When it was a piece of prime rib, only the thickest cut would do. I'd pile a baked potato high with butter and sour cream, bacon and chives, and saturate my salads with extra blue cheese and anchovy dressing. As the weekend progressed, knowing I'd be going back on a diet when Monday dawned, I'd have to eat everything I promised myself I'd never eat again: thick-crust double sausage pizza; French fries and bacon cheeseburgers (half-pounders only); fat kosher hot dogs with big dill pickles and salty potato chips dipped in Coca-Cola; hot fudge sundaes with peppermint ice cream; strawberry cheesecake; fried chicken and mashed potatoes; and barbecued spareribs (never baby backs—they were too lean) with cole slaw and baked beans. I'd only be satisfied when it culminated on Sunday night with a Chinese meal fit for Chairman Mao. A 10-pound gain over a weekend was not uncommon.

It was a toss-up as to who got the bulk of my salary—the grocer, the restaurants or the pharmacy. Despite my enormous appetite, I'd say the pharmacy was the winner. I was taking 10 grams of Synthroid (thyroid medication) and four Lasix (diuretics) daily. Add to that one to two diet pills, mood equalizers, tranquilizers and laxatives. I knew the pills were killing me, but without them my weight gains doubled.

Finally, certain that it was a major malfunction in my body and not my eating habits that caused me to balloon the way I did, I convinced a doctor to put me in the hospital to find out why I was overweight. After three days and a battery of tests, including a full endocrinology work-up, I was pronounced incurably fat. Accompanying that diagnosis was word of a nonfunctioning thyroid, an almost nonfunctioning pituitary and lousy adrenals. I would be on medication the remainder of my life. I was doomed to have a bulbous body forever.

BORN-AGAIN SKINNY

It took an accident and the loving gesture of a friend to change my life. Six months after my fat-for-life diagnosis, I went on a ski trip. On the very first run, I collided violently with a tree, and I woke up in the hospital with a broken leg.

As I lay there on the hospital bed wondering if all I had heard about hospital food was true, I discovered a book among the get-well cards and gifts. It was a book on nutrition given to me by a thoughtful friend. I dug into it, and for the first time in my life, I learned about food and the role it plays in the health of the human body.

I found that my body—like all our bodies—is simply a product of what fuels it. The key is in how we feed this physical machine. We are what we eat, pure and simple. How we look, how we feel, the quality and quantity of our energy, and our health are contingent upon our diets. Food makes our bodies healthy or unhealthy, thin or fat. Food becomes nutrients: vitamins, minerals, amino acids, glucose, lipids and water. If our physical bodies were broken down and put into a test tube, we'd be nothing more than a combination of these nutrients.

As I lay in bed with time to kill, I also took the time to listen to my body. I took the first tentative steps toward breaking through the pills, the guilt and the fat, to actually feel my own body again.

The more I learned about myself, the more I needed to know about nutrition. I devoured everything I could read on the subject, which unfortunately wasn't a lot. This was in the mid-1970s, when a holistic approach to health and nutrition was new to our country. Health food stores were the size of walk-in closets, and the selection of leading-edge nutrition literature was limited to a handful of authors. Even in avant-garde Los Angeles, those few authors were labeled as weirdos, charlatans and health food faddists. I sought out information wherever I could find it as I searched for doctors, nutritionists and health specialists.

Slowly, I weaned myself from the pills. I found healthful foods to replace my beloved junk foods. There was no deprivation, no sacrifice. I still indulged; I just celebrated my newfound knowledge by making better choices. I took responsibility for what I ate and how I ate. I took control of my own body. And I lost weight.

Each ounce shed was victory. Every pound lost was a battle won. Slowly, I edged into slimhood and respectability. I watched not just my weight, but also my sense of well-being. Each morning I awoke feeling better, and each morning I recommitted to my quest to learn more about food and myself, to find out how to feel my body again. I knew I was on the right path. I was keeping off the weight I'd lost. But I still had a long "weigh" to go.

Getting in touch with my body brought new insights into why I gained and lost weight. Learning about nutrition stirred my curiosity, and a healthy skepticism grew. Everything I had learned about food, about nutrition and fat was wrong. And soon I realized that diets—all diets—were wrong, too. Not only did they not work, they weren't healthy. I was looking for much more than a diet. I was looking for a way of eating.

It was then that I stumbled across a book about enzymes and the digestive system called *Food Combining Made Easy* by Herbert Shelton. In it the author suggested that the key to good digestion was in the combination of foods eaten and explained how enzymes played a crucial role in the way our bodies process the nutrients in food.

I dug deeper. As I learned more about digestion and the role of enzymes, I tossed out everything I'd ever been taught about healthy, "balanced" meals. Certainly, we need a balance of protein, carbohydrates and fats, but that balance doesn't come in a single meal or in the artificial three-meals-a-day we somehow have come to consider the "right" way to eat.

Our prehistoric ancestors didn't eat balanced meals. For countless thousands of years, humans' daily regimen of food was controlled by their environment. These wandering omnivores ate from what was at hand. If berries were ripe and plentiful, they ate berries—and they didn't go off in search of tubers and a mammoth to round out the meal.

As our cultures and technologies grew more complex, our eating habits became more a dictate of social and economic forces not beholden to nature or the carefully evolved needs of our bodies. Breakfast, lunch and dinner were more suited to the scheduling needs of factory owners than to the metabolic needs of the factory workers. Once incorporated into our lifestyles over the centuries, the three-squares-a-day approach to eating took on the appearance of normalcy. The "balanced" nutritional needs were compressed into a single meal. And there was the rub. It wasn't "balanced" at all.

I began to develop a way of eating based not on *what* foods I ate, but on what foods I ate *together.* It was the combinations that made the difference. I experimented. Calories were not something to be feared; they were simply units of energy. Weight gain, I discovered, had more to do with efficiency than with fat. How well our body processes the food we eat determines the impact those foods have on our systems—if we gain weight, lose weight or stay the same. Excess fat was a leftover product of the process. Enzymes and combining were the key, and weight loss—permanent lifelong weight loss—was the result.

My weight melted to 98 pounds. (Perhaps a bit too thin, but what fun it was gaining it back!) I was healthy. I was happy. I wasn't afraid of ever being fat again. The guilt was gone, and I could eat anything I wanted.

I began to spread the word, and before I knew it my living room was like the front row at the awards ceremony on Oscar night. My musings on food attracted such celebrity clients as Jack Nicholson, Jodie Foster, Maria Shriver, Liza Minelli, Engelbert Humperdinck, Linda Gray, Marie Osmond, Sally Kellerman, Jennifer Jones, Dick Smothers and others.

The Beverly Hills "Diet Shop" was born. Celebrities, business leaders, housewives and working people were my clients. People who could afford to go anywhere and consult any of the world's experts were consulting with me because they knew I had the answer: I could get them thin.

I became the talk of the town. Calls came from all over the world. Clients traveled cross-country to attend my classes or for private sessions. In response to demand, I wrote a book.

In April 1981, *The Beverly Hills Diet* hit the stores, and the book tour began. Word of Conscious Combining rocketed around the world. I crisscrossed the United Sates innumerable times and was invited to every foreign country in which the book was published, including Japan, South Africa, Australia, Italy, Germany, England, Scotland and Ireland. Over the next two years I visited every continent.

It was toward the end of those whirlwind two years that I felt my message had hit home, and the time had come to slip out of the limelight and go back to simple day-to-day living. I continued with my private consultations, never dreaming that someday I would write *The New Beverly Hills Diet*. I never thought there would be the need. I thought I had said it all.

Born-Again Skinny

Undaunted by the passing years and the stacks of new diets replacing it on the bookshelves around the world, *The Beverly Hills Diet* lived on.

May 1993

> *To Whom It May Concern:*
> *I'm in a desperate search for a few copies of* The Beverly Hills Diet *by Judy Mazel. I have searched every library and bookstore in Chicago and New York to no avail.*
> *I first purchased the book in 1983 after my honeymoon cruise. Ten years later, both my ex-husband and I still faithfully use* The Beverly Hills Diet *to maintain our original loss and shed those few extra pounds we have a tendency to gain over the winter. After six to eight copies between two families, we've finally done it: only one very tattered copy remains. We now circulate a computer chart designed by my ex-husband of*

*the general diet (fortunately for me, I got custody
of the one remaining copy of the book), but the
chart in no way gives us the strength and enthusiasm of the book.*

—Sylvia B.

September 1993
    Dear Judy:
    *I'm hoping you can tell me where I might obtain
a copy of* The Beverly Hills Diet. *I used it 12 to 15
years ago, and it was very effective. I shall appreciate anything you can do to help me locate the
best diet I ever used that worked.*

—Mary S.

September 1994
    Sirs:
    I'm presently re-reading The Beverly Hills Diet
*by Judy Mazel. In the past 12 years, many more
diet books have been written, probably none better than Ms. Mazel's as to results.*

—Mrs. H.

April 1994
    Dear Ms. Mazel:
    *I hope you are still there because I want you to
know how much* The Beverly Hills Diet *has meant
to me. I'm 63 years old and for years hadn't been
able to button my skirts no matter what I did.
Nothing worked. I lost my 10 extra pounds on
your diet, and that was three years ago. I'm so
grateful to you.*

—Terry

The letters kept piling up; the Skinny converts continued losing weight, and new calls for help kept coming, their cries of desperation loud and clear. But diet times had changed. It had become big business.

Today, if you walk into any shopping mall, you'll see that the diet and nutrition sections of bookstores have grown far beyond proportion, as have the shoppers that crowd the aisles. My once high weight of 180 pounds, considered huge by any standards for a woman in 1981, has become commonplace. Lane Bryant, the original "fat" store, has been pushed aside by the mob of competitors attracted to this "expanding" market. Even top designers like Liz Claiborne have jumped on the "fat" bandwagon.

It seems that despite all the medical research, the constant barrage from the media and the proliferation of low- and no-fat foods (a record number of 965 new ones hit the market in 1995), America keeps getting fatter. People who have never previously had a weight problem, who have never been on a diet before, are caught on a treadmill of endless and conflicting advice. Their cries for help, their frustration, their desperation and exasperation are growing daily. Obesity has become a primary health hazard, and it's no wonder. The current crop of diet books can be summed up as "more of the same," as the same recycled fallacies continue to reappear in diet literature. Turn the pages of any of the current crop of diet books, and four themes predominate:

1. The low-fat theme
2. The high-protein, anti-carbohydrate theme

3. The high-carbohydrate, anti-protein theme
4. The psychological theme, i.e., identifying the reasons why you are fat

Certainly books trumpeting the first three themes can be marketed as having the potential to effect weight loss, although all studies—and common sense—will confirm that such weight loss is temporary and unhealthy. Again, I would remind you that 98 percent of all dieters gain their initial weight loss back, and then some, within a year. You simply cannot live a healthy or happy life eating no fat, no protein and/or no carbohydrates. It is the proper balance of all nutrients that keeps you slim and healthy, and the proper balance of foods from all food groups that is going to keep you fit and vibrant. That balance, by the way, as set by the U.S. Senate Committee on Nutrition and Human Needs in its "Dietary Goals for the United States," is 55 to 60 percent carbohydrates, 20 to 25 percent protein and 20 percent unsaturated fats. The study further indicates that the balance need not be filled on a daily basis, but rather on a weekly basis.

Granted, books that take the reader into his or her psyche to understand the conscious and subconscious motivations for overeating may be a good thing, but they don't take the weight off, nor do they stop the overeating. Just because you discover that as a child you ate when your mother failed to acknowledge your achievements—and you are still following that pattern as an adult interacting with other people—doesn't mean that you'll now stop overeating or miraculously shed those extra pounds.

As I said in the introduction, the "why" you eat isn't important. It simply doesn't matter.

What does matter is that in all the years since the publication of *The Beverly Hills Diet,* other than the books that copied or modified my original method of Conscious Combining, no one else has come up with *any new answers.* This includes the medical and scientific communities, who continue to tout their tried and "untrue" methods: pills, powders, calorie counting, exercise, heredity and the elusive fat genes.

Like the hopeful dieters they advise, these experts are caught up in a never-ending cycle of failures and new promises. Each January is a rehash of the previous January as the talk shows and tabloids devote an inordinate amount of time and space to what they term the "answer" to keeping our New Year's resolutions about weight loss. This shameless parade of experts includes gynecologists posing as nutritional experts and chiropractors who have become Doctors of Sports Medicine recommending to people carrying 100 extra pounds that they "joyfully" walk up and down stairs for 40 minutes. Or, better still, telling us how much fun it will be to go to a restaurant and order anything we want right off the menu as long as we tell the waiter to only serve half the portion and pack the other half in a doggie bag. As if any of those doggie bags will *really* make it home. Maybe the bag will find its way home, but the contents will surely be gone, eaten before the hapless, hopeless and hungry dieter even turns the key in the ignition to start the car.

I wonder how many dieters keep their New Year's weight loss resolutions. I'll wager the ONLY resolution

they keep is the new one they make—*to never go on
another diet!* And rightly so.

Diets just don't work. Behavior modification doesn't
work. "Diet shops" don't work. Programs insisting
that you change your lifestyle and habits don't work.
Conscious Combining, the technique I pioneered in
1981, is still the only answer.

Not too long ago, I assessed my continually growing coterie of ever-slim Conscious Combiners and
saw happy, successful Skinnies in a world filled with
hopelessly fat failures. It was devastating. I knew the
time had come to reenter the diet fray, to once again
stick my head out above the crowd and tell the world
about my tried-and-true, *improved* techniques of
Conscious Combining.

You see, I too have grown. Not in size . . . I haven't
slipped back to my old fatty ways. I'm still the same
slim person I was in 1981. But I have grown in
knowledge, in the practical, livable application of the
techniques I pioneered. My years of continual experimentation have confirmed what I had so unabash-
edly boasted on national TV. I have indeed "discovered
the cure for fat."

True, I stepped out of the limelight years ago. But
I continued in private practice, and my lifestyle
remained relatively unchanged. Through six world
cruises and a year of living abroad; through days and
nights filled with the finest dining on varieties of
international cuisine; through constant rounds of
charity balls, ladies' luncheons, social brunches,
business lunches and constant travel, I have kept
close tabs on my rapidly expanding (in numbers, not

girth) international clientele. I accumulated copious notes that have been a priceless reference as I refined and fine-tuned my original rules. Rules that haven't changed dramatically (you can't change the physical laws that govern the human body), but that I have adjusted to make them more livable. My goal was to make *The New Beverly Hills Diet* not a diet, but rather a lifestyle eating program that included weight loss and maintenance—a "weigh of life" for the 1990s and a new "diet consciousness."

Diet times have changed and so have the diet-conscious. As the failures and foibles of "dieting" have been uncovered, many are now realizing that food deprivation and denial aren't the answer. Exposed to the fallacies of the no-fat, low-fat, high-protein, anti-carbohydrate, anti-protein, high-carbohydrate diet regimes, perennial dieters are healing the scars of fad dieting. They are waiting, hoping and praying for something new. Well . . . I have that something new . . . the lifestyle eating plan that is, indeed, everyone's dream come true!

In the years since the development and publication of my original book, *The Beverly Hills Diet*, I learned that it is not necessary to go on a lengthy 42-day regimen that focuses primarily on fruit, or to begin with 10 days of nothing but fruit. I learned that abstaining from eating animal protein for 18 days, as was the case in my original diet, also isn't necessary.

While the role of the enzymes in the specific fruits remains critical, as does the combination of foods eaten, the non-mixing of food groups does not have to be so restrictive and unrelenting. In fact, with the aid of these natural enzymes and the application of my technique of "Conscious Compensation," we can mix quite frequently without suffering any of the negative side effects . . . added pounds or impaired health and vitality.

In an ideal world, the less we mix food groups, the better off we'll be. Unfortunately, we don't live in an ideal world, we live in reality. And reality means eating the foods and combinations of foods we've grown accustomed to eating: meat loaf and mashed potatoes, biscuits and gravy, a burger with fries, turkey and all the fixin's. I've learned that with the implementation of Conscious Combining, coupled with my now more highly developed technique of Conscious Compensation, this style of reality eating is not only possible, it's preferable. Preferable because it's reality! And the growing legions of my forever-slim Conscious Combiners are the proof in the pudding.

My only dilemma was how to effectively transmit my new message. Simply writing another book wasn't the answer. Dieters are interested in only one thing: losing weight! And invariably the only chapter in diet books that captures their attention is the "diet" chapter. The rest of the book gets little, if any, attention. My years of interaction with an untold number of my readers—the unsuccessful as well as the successful—confirmed that it had to be something more, something that would offer a more powerful support system. It had to be something they couldn't just skim through, something that would engender confidence and commitment and that could have the same effect on a group or a single person. It was a seemingly impossible task to accomplish in the form of a traditional chapter-by-chapter book.

Further, I realized that lifestyle and eating changes don't happen chapter by chapter, but rather day by day. One of the reasons people who attend my classes or seminars are so successful is because they receive a boost of support each day while they are on the program. Achieving this same interactive feeling in book form wouldn't be easy.

Inasmuch as making successful Skinnies, not selling books, was my goal, I began building a solution one step at a time. Step one . . . *The New Beverly Hills Diet Slimkit.* Consisting of four audiocassettes and the *Little Skinny Book,* it is a hand-holding guide that allows me to talk people through the 35-day program. The very same audio program has been adapted and incorporated into this book, as well as being available on its own.

Not a diet but a lifestyle eating program, *The New Beverly Hills Diet Slimkit* confirmed that you don't have to wait to lose weight before you can eat the foods you love. Day 1 begins not only with fruit, but with "real" food. A new way to eat, enjoy and lose weight, the 35-day program includes 21 wide-open meals to indulge food fantasies.

Launched on one of the premier shopping channels, *The New Beverly Hills Diet Slimkit* followed in the footsteps of its predecessor, *The Beverly Hills Diet,* by breaking sales records. Over the next two years, I continued hands-on testing across the country, not with movie stars and celebrities as I had with the original diet, but with real people living regular lives.

It soon became clear that tapes alone weren't enough. They left dieters needing something visual to refer back to. I discovered that this lack of an easy reference impeded the development of a full understanding of my concept. So it was back to the drawing board until, at last, the dream came true— the birth of *The New Beverly Hills Diet.*

The book that has it all: a day-by-day diary preceded by a conventionally formatted book with a full explanation of the program. Augment this book with the audiocassette program, *The New Beverly Hills Diet Slimkit,* and CyberSkinny, my interactive World Wide Web site (http://www.cyberskinny.com), and you have the whole enchilada. (Oh, yes, enchiladas are on the diet, too.)

This time you can't help but win . . . or should I say lose!

Enzyme Your Weigh to Ecstasy

Food is pleasure. Food is guilt. Food is reward. Food is also the raw material and fuel that build and power your body. You are what you eat, pure and simple. The well-being of our bodies is dependent on the food we supply. It is our choice. No one forces us to eat anything. We pick the time. We pick the place. We choose the food that will become us; the food that will be converted into the flesh, bone, blood and, yes, the fat that make up our bodies.

With that in mind, let me get to the heart of Conscious Combining: It isn't *what* you eat or *how much* you eat that makes you fat; it is *when* you eat and *what you eat together!*

This is nothing new. The principles of Conscious Combining on which *The New Beverly Hills Diet* is based go back thousands of years. The first recorded discussion of these principles was in China's *Classics of Internal Medicine of the Yellow Emperor* (2598-1606 B.C.), but the principles had clearly been known for centuries before. Food combining was widely practiced in ancient times—particularly in China and ancient Persia—and the practice has persisted right up to our century, when it was primarily the province of health faddists, as they were called.

The principles of food combining are dictated by what happens during the digestive process. The purpose of digestion, of course, is to turn food into the nutrients that sustain life: carbohydrates provide energy; proteins become the building blocks of flesh, bone and blood; fat acts as a transport medium for vitamins and hormones, while lecithin, a fatty acid, is an emulsifier and a key constituent of the sheath that surrounds our nerve cells.

As I said earlier, the process of digestion begins with and is contingent upon enzymes. These biological catalysts are in the food we eat and are also activated in our bodies by the food we eat.

There are four stages in the digestive process: (1) digestion; (2) absorption; (3) metabolism; and (4) elimination.

THE DIGESTIVE PROCESS

STAGE 1: DIGESTION

Food's first stop in the body is your mouth, and that's where digestion begins. Initiated by chewing and found in the alkaline juices of saliva, an enzyme called *ptyalin* starts the breakdown of carbohydrates. Ptyalin does not act on proteins, fats and fruits (a special category of carbohydrates), all of which continue unaffected to the next stage, your stomach.

If a carbohydrate has been properly digested by ptyalin, it is already in the form of a crystalline sugar called maltose by the time it reaches your stomach. In the stomach, maltose is further broken down before it moves on to the next stage.

The stomach is also where proteins are digested. The process begins as hydrochloric acid attacks the fat and activates the enzyme *pepsin.* As the hydrochloric acid and other substances convert the fat to lipids, the pepsin softens and begins to break down the protein into amino acids. Next, the hydrochloric acid and pepsin work in concert to complete the reduction of protein into amino acids.

By the time proteins, carbohydrates and fats reach the next stop, your small intestine, they have already been turned into nutrients.

Fruits, however, are carbohydrates in a class of their own. To be digested, they have no need of your body's enzymes; fruits already contain all of the enzymes necessary to reduce them to nutrients. They pass unscathed through your mouth and stomach until, in the small intestine, the fruits' enzymes act to convert them to nutrients. Because of their eminent digestibility, fruits move quickly through your system. Before you've barely finished your last bite of fruit, the first bite's nutrients are entering your bloodstream.

STAGE 2: ABSORPTION

It is at this stage that food's nutrients, including water-soluble vitamins and minerals, enter the bloodstream. Through the bloodstream they are distributed throughout your body to nourish your cells.

STAGE 3: METABOLISM

Metabolism is the engine that powers and maintains our bodies. This is the stage at which nutrients, the proteins, are transformed into the building materials that create and replenish our flesh, bone and blood. It is here that we "fuel up" with the energy carbohydrates provide. And it is here that we begin to feel—for good or ill—the effects of what we eat. Contrary to what you may think, there is no such thing as a slow metabolism. You control your own metabolism and metabolic rate through your eating habits.

STAGE 4: ELIMINATION

This last stage is where the by-products of the nutrients, the waste products your body doesn't need, are discarded. It is a constant process involving respiration, perspiration and excretion through urination and bowel movements.

Each stage of the digestive process is subject to the effects of what you eat. Mix the relatively fast, alkaline-medium process of carbohydrate breakdown with the rather slow, acid-medium process of protein breakdown, and the digestive system is utterly confounded.

If you eat an apple all by itself, it will be processed through your stomach in some 15 to 20 minutes; an enzymatic fruit such as papaya will take even less time.

If you eat a protein meal—shrimp and steak, for example—it will remain in your system for upwards of four or five hours. Eat the apple or papaya on an empty stomach at the start of the day, and it moves unfettered from the stomach into the small intestine. Eat the fruit after the shrimp and steak, however, and it remains blocked in the stomach by the protein. Eat a steak and baked potato and the carbohydrate enzyme needed to digest the potato will be neutralized by the protein enzymes.

But inefficient digestion—indigestion—is more than heartburn; likewise, it's more than just ineffective in terms of nutrition. We all have experienced the effects of less than optimum nutrition. Lack of energy, nervous tension, depression, and dull hair and skin are all potentially the result of indigestion. We have also felt the pain, bloating, discomfort, gas or stomach ache it can produce. But how many of us realize that our added fat, or extra pounds, is a product of our digestion gone awry? FAT (OR ADDED POUNDS) IS JUST ANOTHER SYMPTOM OF INDIGESTION.

If our bodies broke down food the way they should, absorbed and metabolized all that they should in the way that they should, and if, in turn, they eliminated the waste, then *nothing would be left over.* We could not gain weight. We could not get fat. The presence of those added pounds means that one or more of the four stages of the digestive process—digestion, absorption, metabolism and elimination—have not occurred efficiently.

In the case of carbohydrates, this can occur if they move through that first stage of digestion—the mouth—without being acted on by ptyalin. Your system is geared up to process maltose, so when the wayward carbohydrate hits your stomach, there it stays, well on its way to fat.

How can you make sure that the first stage of carbohydrate digestion is effective? There are three rules for moving carbohydrates successfully through your digestive system to make them nonfattening and energy producing. Contrary to what you have been hearing, you DO NOT have to give them up; you simply have to:

1. *Chew your food.* I hate to sound like your mother, but she was right. Chewing triggers ptyalin and masticates the food to fully expose it to the enzyme. So go ahead, luxuriate in eating that flavorful mouthful. Just chew, chew, chew!
2. *Beware of sweeteners.* It's the sugar in the baked goods, not the fat, that makes *you* fat. Whenever you mix sweeteners with a grain, such as flour or corn meal, the combination neutralizes the ptyalin and you end up with a stomach full of undigested carbohydrates.
3. *Avoid mixing carbohydrates with proteins or eating carbohydrates after proteins.* With proteins: carbohydrates do not require as much digesting time in your stomach as proteins. However, when they are eaten with proteins, they become trapped. After proteins: hydrochloric acid and pepsin are activated when a fatty protein reaches your stomach. The hydrochloric acid breaks down the fat and activates the pepsin so it can begin its work. When these enzymes act together, they create an acid medium that neutralizes ptyalin, inhibiting full carbohydrate digestion.

Your body digests proteins slowly; hence, once they enter your digestive system, your body will be unable to digest carbohydrates for the remainder of the cycle. You can expect meat to remain in an efficient stomach for up to 10 hours; poultry about 7 hours; fish 6. Bear in mind that most of us do not have efficient digestive systems and the process may take considerably longer.

What can you do to ensure that your body efficiently digests the foods you feed it? That's the point of Conscious Combining. For starters, you can take charge of how your body processes nutrients by making conscious choices about the types of foods you eat and when you eat them. You'll be learning how to do that on the 35-day Born-Again Skinny program you'll soon be starting.

Critical to the success of Conscious Combining is the technique of enhancing the enzymatic action in your body through the use of the natural enzymes in certain very specific fruits—the same fruits you'll be eating on the program.

I must admit that I'm confounded by the total lack of research addressing enzymes and body weight. True, the science of enzymology is of recent origin. Enzymes were only first "discovered" in 1878, and it was 1926 before an enzyme was crystallized in the laboratory. While the determination of enzymatic sequences dates only to 1967, and enzymes continue to be identified and their effects traced to this day, it seems that the thrust of enzyme research thus far has been on exploring the potential for disease therapies and genetic engineering, not weight loss.

However, it has been 15 years since I pioneered the

idea of body fat, or added weight as the case may be, as a product of indigestion and enzymatic action in *The Beverly Hills Diet*. Quick to follow my example, a stream of other lay authors adopted my ideas as they explored the relationship between enzymes, simple food combining and weight loss. In the intervening years, while anecdotal evidence has mounted with each successful adherent to my principles of Conscious Combining, there still have been no controlled scientific studies to finally bring discussion of this theory into the scientific mainstream. Though they have been quick to criticize and disavow the theory, I fear that the mighty nutritional dogma of the medical community keeps the "experts" from uncovering or even asking the question: "Why does it work?"

Let me state it again, loudly and clearly: It is not food that causes weight gain, it is inefficiently digested food. The major cause of inefficient digestion is the overburdening of the digestive system through eating too many different kinds of foods together at the same time. The imbalance of the balanced meal!

Somewhere around the middle of the 20th century, in prosperous and advanced societies like ours, it became possible to obtain virtually any food at virtually any season of the year. The "balanced meal" was held up as an icon for a thriving "modern" culture enjoying a booming economy. And eating three times a day was infinitely more practical than eating "whenever." Technologies of food preservation were refined and perfected, then taken a step further to prompt the actual creation of new foods altogether—wholly artificial or "junk" foods, touted as another important time-saver for a democracy on the move. And obesity became one of the new diseases of the age (see chapter 6).

What the "balanced meal" failed to account for is the way the digestive process works. If you combine food groups, you not only make it harder for the enzymes to do their job—again, enzymes for one food group cannot "cross over" to work on other food groups—you also actually impede enzymatic action.

I ask you, if the traditional balanced meal worked, would 60 million Americans be fat?

The New Beverly Hills Diet makes use of the facts of digestion and enzymatic action to let the individual plan eating experiences—or to "work around" the facts if the plan cannot be met—by paying attention to food combinations and to when the combinations are eaten. *This is the essence of Conscious Combining.* It enables the individual not only to stop miscombining, but to combine proactively for efficient digestion that rids the body of toxins, ensures energy and maintains slimhood on a lifelong basis.

That means that if you know that a dinner party is coming up or if it's Thanksgiving next week or if you could not resist going out for brunch, you can plan for, or around, those events. And if you indulge in more miscombinations than your digestive system can tolerate, if you "binge," you then turn to another feature of the program, Conscious Compensation, to apply corrective counterparts.

FOOD GROUPS

To fully understand Conscious Combining, we must be aware of the types of foods we eat and how our bodies will process them. As we have discussed, proteins, carbohydrates and fats form the three major food groups, with a half-protein, half-carbohydrate subgroup comprised primarily of legumes, the either/or's.

All foods contain at least one, or more of these nutrients, and most foods contain all of them to varying degrees. How we classify a food according to group is dependent upon the major component of the food. If 51 percent or more of a food is made up of glucose, it is considered a carbohydrate; if 51 percent or more is amino acids, it is a protein; and if 51 percent or more is lipids, it is a fat.

Experts agree that 55 to 60 percent of our daily calories should come from carbohydrates, with fats contributing 20 percent and proteins adding the remaining 20 to 25 percent.

Proteins

Beef	Kefir	Pork	Desserts:
Cheese	Lamb	Seafood	Cheesecake
Eggs	Milk	Seeds	Crème brûlée
Fish	Nuts	Yogurt	Crème caramel
Fowl	Nut butters		Flan
			Ice cream

Fats

Butter	Mayonnaise	Sour cream
Heavy cream	Oil	Whipped cream

Carbohydrates

Fruits

(a carb in a
  category all
  it's own)
All fruits
Brandy
Champagne
Cognac
Wine

50/50—
Either/Or

Avocados
Garbanzo beans
Kidney beans
Lentils
Lima beans
Peanuts
Pinto beans
Soybeans

Mini-
Carbohydrates

Asparagus
Celery
Crookneck squash
Herbs
Kale
Lettuce
Mushrooms
Mustard greens
Parsley
Zucchini

Midi-
Carbohydrates

Beets
Broccoli
Brussels sprouts
Cabbage
Carrots
Cauliflower
Cucumbers
Eggplant
Leeks
Onions
Parsnips
Peas
Peppers (red,
  green and chile)
Radishes
Shallots
String beans
Tomatoes
Turnips

Maxi-
Carbohydrates

Artichokes
Barley
Breads
Buckwheat
Bulgur
Cake (white,
  sponge, choc-
  olate, carrot)
Chocolate
Cookies
Corn
Cornmeal
Couscous
Cream of Wheat
Farina
Grains
Millet
Oatmeal
Oats
Pasta
Pie crust
Potatoes
Rice
Rye
Wheat
Winter Squash

Alcohol:
  Beer
  All distilled:
    Bourbon, Rum,
    Scotch, Tequila,
    Vodka, etc.

Proteins are the most difficult foods to digest because they require as many as 12 steps before they completely break down into nutrients.

Of the proteins, dairy products are the slowest to digest. High in fat and low in moisture, they present a difficult challenge for digestion.

The complexity of carbohydrates dictates how much time they take to digest, with the most complex carbohydrates, the maxi-carbohydrates, taking the longest. A maxi such as a potato will take some three hours to digest, while a mini-carbohydrate such as a mushroom will take only an hour.

One carbohydrate is not more fattening than another. Mini, midi or maxi . . . all carbohydrates yield the same four calories per gram regardless of the complexity of their molecular structure.

Fats are almost never eaten alone, so we really don't need to know how they act alone in our digestive systems. On the minus side, they slow down digestion. On the plus side, fats do not interfere with any enzymatic actions and can be combined with a carbohydrate or a protein, but not a fruit (nothing really combines with fruit).

Fruits digest the fastest of all foods, hence they can be combined with **no other foods.** Moving through your stomach in no more than an hour when eaten alone, fruits will be trapped in your stomach by any slower foods that join them.

CONSCIOUS COMBINING

The essential principles of Conscious Combining are easy to remember and easy to follow. With time, adhering to the principles becomes routine.

1. Ideally, proteins go with proteins; carbohydrates go with carbohydrates; fruit must be eaten alone.
2. Begin each day with a single enzymatic fruit from the list of fruits included in the 35-day weight loss plan—i.e., pineapple, strawberries, grapes, papaya, watermelon, mango, kiwi, persimmon, prunes, apricots or figs.

   You may eat as much of the fruit as you want, but eat just one fruit at a time—don't mix grapes with strawberries, for example.

   Wait one hour before switching from one fruit to another fruit.

   Wait two hours before eating food from another food group.

   Once you eat food from another food group, do not eat fruit again for the remainder of the day.
3. If the next food you eat after fruit is a carbohydrate, you may eat them without restriction until you eat a protein.
4. Once you eat protein, no matter how small the amount—even if it is just milk in your coffee or chicken in your Caesar salad—80 percent of what you eat for the balance of the day *should* be protein.
5. Carbohydrates are carbohydrates—whether starch, vegetables, salads, cereals or grains— and, *for the most part,* they should not be combined with protein.
6. Proteins are proteins—whether meat, fish, milk,

yogurt, cheese, nuts, seeds or ice cream—and, *for the most part,* they should not be combined with carbohydrates.

7. Fats such as butter, oil, mayonnaise, sour cream and heavy cream can be combined with either proteins or carbohydrates, but **not** with fruit.

8. Eliminate diet sodas, artificial sweeteners, diet products containing artificial sweeteners and artificial additives, nondairy creamer and margarine. Limit, if not eliminate, any foods with artificial additives (see chapter 6).

9. Most alcoholic beverages are carbohydrates (beer, bourbon, rum, vodka, scotch, tequila) and should, for the most part, be consumed only with carbohydrates; wine is a fruit and can be combined with other fruits; *champagne is neutral and goes with anything.*

Unlike the rash of other "diet" methods popularized over the years, Conscious Combining is not restrictive. It's liberating! These easy-to-follow principles offer the flexibility to eat all kinds of food and all kinds of meals. I can't stress this single point strongly enough. **If all you do is follow the second principle and begin each and every day with a single enzymatic fruit, you'll maintain your lost weight even if you eat one "open" meal every day.**

Conscious Combining is a way of planning what you'll eat during the course of a day and adjusting your plan as the day progresses. For example, if you assume that dinner is going to be your "open" meal— the meal in which you combine carbohydrates and proteins by eating, say, a hamburger and French fries—you would plan to eat only carbohydrates for lunch and snacks that day (following your morning fruit, of course). But if you change the plan and eat a burger and fries for lunch instead, you must eat primarily protein for the rest of the day; that means dinner might be steak or shrimp, or both, accompanied by a small amount of a carbohydrate. (Remember the 80 percent protein rule.)

CONSCIOUS COMPENSATION

Another reason that this is a program for lifelong slimhood is that it offers ways to recoup from too much miscombining. With Conscious Compensation, you consume specific foods to counteract the effects of the miscombinations. These correctives can be eaten either after the fact or, if you know in advance that you are going to miscombine, before the fact.

ANTIDOTES TO BE EATEN FOR BREAKFAST THE DAY AFTER

1. Greasy, creamy, cheesy foods (e.g., pizza, Mexican food, ice-cream binge, fried chicken, spareribs and fries):
   Burn with pineapple or strawberries.
2. Protein overdose (e.g., prime rib, steak, barbecue):
   Soften and digest with papaya or mango (papaya after meat, mango after fowl).
3. Sweets (e.g., cake, cookies and candy):
   Scrub with grapes.

4. Salt overdose:
   Wash with watermelon or mop with meat.

PRECEDOTES TO BE EATEN FOR BREAKFAST THE DAY YOU KNOW YOU ARE GOING TO BE EATING THE FOLLOWING

1. Greasy, creamy, cheesy foods:
   Precede with pineapple or strawberries.
2. Salty foods:
   Breakfast on dried apricots.

When Conscious Compensation offers more than one corrective choice, time and testing will determine what works best for you. For example, if you experience excessive bloating after a salty meal and watermelon doesn't work—that is, if you don't lose the weight you gained—try an all-meat day instead. If that does the trick, you'll know that protein is your bloat antidote.

A Medical Doctor's Opinion

I'm a specialist in Internal Medicine. I have been in practice in Beverly Hills, California, for 35 years. What Judy Mazel has discovered has been a truly eye-opening experience.

In the days of my training as an internist, the professors taught the standard nutritional theory. That theory states that you count the calories you eat in a day and subtract what you burn, and that tells you whether you gained or lost weight. This is a problem because it doesn't seem to hold true in all patients. This was always somewhat confusing to me. Then I read a book by Judy Mazel called *The Beverly Hills Diet*. Judy explained the mystery in simple terms. I realized she wrote the book for lay people, but I assure you as a medical doctor that the approach is perfectly correct.

In medical school we take a course called biochemistry. In biochemistry, we learn about a critical metabolic cycle called the Krebs cycle. This is the underlying metabolic cycle that relates to calorie

storage. Scientists named it after the doctor who discovered it and the citric acid cycle that is the entry
point into this cycle.

The cycle is as follows: Proteins are broken down
into tiny molecules called amino acids. Fats are broken down into small molecules such as acetoacetic
acids. Carbohydrates are broken down into small
metabolic acids such as citric acid. This explains how
the body stores calories. The body stores excess calories in the cells of the body and this leads to obesity.
What technique can we use to prevent excess calories
from going through the citric acid cycle and being
stored in cells as energy far beyond the need of the
cell? In other words, how can we prevent obesity?
This is especially important to answer since we eat
proteins, carbohydrates and fats every day, and frequently all in the same meal. It is my opinion that
Judy Mazel made the fundamental discovery.

The basic discovery was Conscious Combining. By
that we mean putting foods together that digest
together. It means avoiding those foods that ferment
and cause calorie retention. All of you who have read
The Beverly Hills Diet remember Judy's basic rules:
Proteins go with other proteins and fats. Carbs go
with other carbs and fats. Fruit goes alone. Fats go
with either proteins or carbohydrates. By following
these simple rules and the sample menus that Judy
gives you, you'll find that you'll lose weight by doing
things that seem impossible to chronic dieters.

You'll lose weight eating potato pancakes. You'll lose
weight eating bagels. You'll lose weight eating pizza.
You'll lose weight eating baked potatoes. You'll lose
weight eating a hamburger with everything on it, or

steak, lobster, eggs and toast. You'll lose weight eating popcorn. You'll be able to have Chinese, Japanese or Middle Eastern dinners and still lose weight.

I realize that this is shocking to people who have been yo-yo dieting their entire lives. However, by proper Conscious Combining, you'll be able to eat all of these foods and more, and still lose weight.

Just as important, while you are doing this, you are not on pills or medication. You also will be insuring a lifelong slimhood with good health and great eating. Eating will again be a pleasure and not something of which you are fearful.

I would like to add a medical summary relating to weight reduction. We all know that vanity is the driving force in most cases for weight reduction. We want to look good and be able to fit into our clothes.

However, there are some very sound medical reasons for weight reduction. To begin with, diabetes is very common in overweight people, especially middle-aged people. Long before insulin was discovered, dietary manipulation was the only treatment for diabetes. I guarantee if you are a mild diabetic taking medication for diabetes, weight reduction will provide a cure.

Obesity can also contribute to hypertension. Many people lower the dose or stop taking blood pressure medication completely after they lose weight. Maintaining your ideal weight also substantially improves gout. Obese people tend to be much higher surgical risks than thin people. This is true for any kind of surgery, but especially where surgery requires general anesthesia.

When I first discovered *The Beverly Hills Diet,* I was

a bit skeptical. However, I followed the diet plan and found that while I was eating excellent food, I still lost weight. I then did the literary research that enabled me to understand what Conscious Combining really means in medical and biochemical terms. I found *The Beverly Hills Diet* to be a superb program. This new book promises to be even more satisfying.

I have told you the medical reasons for keeping down your weight. Judy Mazel has struck upon a method where food can be a pleasure and the total calorie consumption is not the issue with which you are dealing. Instead, you are using Conscious Combining and eating the proper mixture of foods.

By doing this, you'll look good, you'll feel good, and you'll be grateful to Judy Mazel.

I wish you well and hope that you follow Judy's diet method.

Albert Sokol, M.D.

Reality

Animals know enough to eat what is under the rock and not the rock itself. Instinctively, our primitive ancestors knew as well. Their pantry was what grew in the grasslands, their bounty came from the forest, their larder was the shore and shallow waters. They harvested plants and animals from nature, and for countless millennia our ancestors' diet was a health-food aficionado's dream. Through generations of trial and error, humans understood what worked and what didn't. But no matter what they ate, it was food, real food, not the rocks. They had no choice.

We have a choice, thousands of choices. A drive down any highway is a journey to fast-food temptation. A stroll down any supermarket aisle is an adventure in snack seduction. Low-fat, no-fat, new, improved, packed, stacked, wrapped and bagged, our food is a never-ending stream of factory fare. It's all designed to woo us gape-jawed into its spell of ease and convenience. It's big business, very big business, and the bank accounts of the purveyors of processed foods are getting bigger and fatter, and so are we!

Of course, we really have no one to blame but ourselves. In spite of all the talk about eating healthier foods, we are eating more chemical-laden, fatter and bigger foods than ever before. If they build it big, we'll come and get it. Where freshness and quality of ingredients were once determining factors in our decision to buy, convenience is what counts now and big is what's really in. Whether it's fast foods, convenience foods, snacks or fancy restaurants, bigger is what sells.

And we are what we eat!

Next time you're at the market, pick up a package of food and read the ingredients. How many names do you recognize? How many names can you even pronounce? Odds are, the ingredient list—if you can even read it—is in such tiny print that it reads like the index of a chemistry text. Is this food? Or is it rocks? Well, I'm here to tell you, it certainly is not food!

Monodiglycerides, sodium nitrate, sodium sorbanate, BHT: chemicals by the pound are poured into the food we eat. And those pounds add to your pounds. How do these compounds affect the natural function of digestion? What are the effects of our increasingly chemical-laden diet? Our scientific and medical communities can't be blind. Just as they can no longer disavow the merits of food combining and the enormous potential of enzymes, they cannot continue to wear blinders as they force-feed us laboratory-made substitutes . . . chemical compounds disguised as food.

Trust me, they know the facts, and the fact is that the human body is not capable of turning chemical additives/artificial foods into nutrients that can be absorbed, metabolized or eliminated. Likewise, these chemical compounds cannot simply pass through our bodies as is; only water and cellulose can do that. Hence, they are absorbed for an indefinite period of time, impeding digestion and adding extra pounds to our weight.

The length of time it takes the human body to ultimately eliminate the pounds of chemicals it is inundated with is unknown. No published scientific studies on the subject are available.

It's interesting to note that preservatives such as sodium nitrate, sodium propinate and BHT are stored in our fat cells. When I suggested to the doctor who informed me of this fact that perhaps this accounted for the difficulty people had in losing weight, his response was, "That's not very scientific!" Maybe it wasn't scientific, but it was good common sense.

The human body runs on nutrients (food) and the food you eat is your choice. It's all up to you. You must take charge. The heart of Conscious Combining and the key to your success as a Born-Again Skinny is taking responsibility for your own body. Don't count on the experts; use your own common sense—it is millions of years in the making. Take charge of what you eat. Think about every bite you put into your body.

Food, as pleasurable as it is, really has a single purpose: to provide our bodies with the raw materials to sustain life. Every bite you take that contains wasted nutrition, every bite you take that contains chemicals, steals from your body. And most of the frozen, packaged or bagged food that you buy is filled with wasted nutrition. From gourmet fare to baby formula to school lunches to fast food, our daily diet of manufactured convenience has become a nutritional nightmare. We must open our eyes. It's time to wake up!

As I've said, *The New Beverly Hills Diet* is a program for lifelong slimhood. This life choice of good nutrition will take some effort at first, but like Conscious Combining, it will soon become second nature. To help you on your way, try to keep these three thoughts in mind when you're grocery shopping:

1. *Be wary of any processed food.* This includes any food that has been cooked. Don't be deluded into thinking that the luscious, unseasoned, "no salt added" cooked chicken in the deli at your local supermarket is what it seems. It was probably not even from the market's own poultry supply. The safe-handling laws in most states would prohibit that. Instead, it came from a poultry purveyor, already soaked in a preserving solution and pre-injected with salt.

2. *Buy the food, not the package!* Don't fall prey to marketing. Think about what's inside the box or bag. After all, it soon will be inside you.

3. *Read the labels.* Be a smart and suspicious shopper. Don't assume something is "fresh" or "healthy" just because the package says it is. Take a close, hard look at the ingredients—*not the percentages, the ingredients.*

And when I say take a close, hard look, I mean a *close, hard* look. On a recent visit to my mother's, I scrutinized her cupboard and was amazed to discover that a box of popular breakfast cereal did not contain any preservatives. Boldly labeled on the box's side panel was a list titled "Ingredients." To my surprise, they were *all natural!* Then I moved on to the "Vitamins and Minerals" list—it told a much different story. A mega-list of vitamins and minerals opened the column, but it ended with BHT—a preservative. Hardly a vitamin or a mineral, it clearly belonged with the ingredients, not hidden away with the vitamins and minerals. And, no, it was not a misprint.

As luck would have it, later that same day I found myself ensconced in an airport shuttle with a lawyer from that same cereal manufacturer. She was headed back to her home after attending a seminar for food industry lawyers held in Chicago.

"What a coincidence!" I exclaimed upon hearing her occupation and place of employment, and I began questioning her about the legality of the misplaced ingredient I'd discovered. She was shocked because it was mislabeled. A year prior to my discovery it was to have been moved from its misleading position on the package to a more appropriate location.

This incident took place on February 5, 1996. I'm sure if you check the more popular brands of breakfast cereals on your grocery shelf, you'll find that this "untruth" in labeling still exists. It does as I write this in the summer of 1996.

Whom can we trust? Whom can we count on? I repeat, it's all up to you. Trust yourself and your own good sense. An important part of learning to take control of what you eat is learning how to eat to live. And that begins with being a smart consumer.

The Skinny Scene

Two things fatten people: their social life and their emotional life. I fall prey to both. Most of us do. Unfortunately, we are members of a food-oriented society. Business meetings take place over breakfast, lunch, cocktails and dinner. We entertain with food. We socialize with food. We celebrate with food. Now, with the popularity of gourmet cooking classes, we love to learn about food, too. One-upmanship these days seems to ride on out-cooking one another. Cooking and eating are our number one pastimes.

Don't worry: to be a Skinny you don't have to give up the joys of either cooking or eating in the company of family, friends and business associates. You'll only have to make a few adjustments, and most of those adjustments will be minor and temporary. There's no longer any reason for you to eat yourself under the table because now there is nothing on that table that you can't have! Whether you are off to a party down the block or on a business trip across the world, you can take your new Skinny eating lifestyle with you.

PARTIES

Parties fool even the most stout-hearted (or should I say slim-hearted?). Traditionally, parties have always represented an opportunity to go crazy: those special occasions when all our excuses are allowed; when everybody is blowing it and no one is watching. But that's the old diet consciousness that says parties are the last supper. From now on, you are going to make them the best of times. And I'm going to help you.

First and foremost, don't make social sacrifices. Don't stay home just because you are on a day where you have to eat something specific. If it is something your host or hostess won't be serving and you don't want to be tempted by other delicious foods, call in advance and explain your situation . . .

We were invited to a friend's house for Super Bowl Sunday. I phoned the hostess and told her I couldn't come. I explained what I was doing. I didn't think I could spend a whole afternoon around all those snacks since I was just supposed to be eating pineapple that day. Then I got to thinking about another friend of ours that would be there. He was a recovering alcoholic. If he could be around everyone drinking all day, certainly I could be happy eating pineapple and drinking champagne. I phoned her back and said we would be there. Well, we went and I didn't

*miss out on a thing except the regret I would have
felt if we hadn't gone. I would have missed out on
all the fun.*

—Nancy, Washington

Give yourself permission to enjoy the party without
guilt or fear. Trust in the program, in the techniques
you are learning and applying, and in yourself. And
when your head says no and your heart says go and
eating is upon you, hang on to those emerging hipbones and just repeat to yourself, "I used to be fat.
I'm not fat anymore and I'll never be fat again!" Then
relax and have fun. You're getting skinny!

It's important to make conscious real-world food
choices from the very beginning. The choice, of
course, can always be to modify any of the days of
the 35-day weight loss program. You'll learn how to
do that once you actually begin. However, if you don't
want to modify, then do what Nancy did: call your
hostess in advance and explain your situation. You
can always offer to bring another dish—one that you
can eat, too.

When I go to a party I keep one thought foremost in
mind when I pass the food: "Is it worth it?" I know
that for every bite of food that goes in my mouth
something else can't. I'm always mindful that what I
choose to eat will determine what I have to eat, and,
what I can't eat later (see chapter 5). Not to mention
that sooner or later I'm going to get full and I won't be
able to fit any more in. Well, I certainly don't want to
be too full to eat something spectacular that's yet to
come because I ate something I didn't even particularly like to begin with.

LITTLE SKINNY PARTY TIPS

Practical Pointers

1. Avoid chips, nuts, pretzels, pickles, cheese, gelatin molds, raw vegetables and dip (unless you are eating only carbohydrates).

2. Do not eat fruit or anything mixed with fruit (beverages included)—unless, of course, you have eaten nothing but fruit up to that point and do not intend to eat anything else for two hours.

3. No mixes other than water or soda with alcoholic beverages.

4. Champagne is the preferred alcoholic beverage.

5. On the day of the party, do not eat any protein until you get to the party. Once the party is over—no matter what time of the day or night it is—if you have eaten protein, 80 percent of what you eat for the balance of the day should be protein.

6. Always purchase your breakfast fruit for the morning after the party in advance, so it is home waiting for you.

7. Weigh yourself every day—no matter what.

Mind over Matter Reminders

- **Don't use your social life as an excuse.** Make a commitment before you go to a party and stick to it. Remember, nobody can make you taste anything. Your social life will go on and there will be many more dinners and many more parties. You won't miss out on anything except a pound or two.

- **Before one morsel passes your lips, check it all out.** Look over the whole spread—everything—including desserts. Then, whatever your choice, enjoy yourself. Just eat like a human being, with one hand, one bite at a time. Always be mindful that *it's not how much you eat in how short a time, it is how long you can make the pleasure last.*

- **Stay on guard.** Simply because the food is there, you are under no obligation to eat it. If you are caught at a party where the food isn't worth eating, and certainly not worth gaining weight for, then carefully pick the foods you eat. Try to be conscious of their category and remember that if you eat protein, you must then steer clear of the carbohydrates.

- **Above all, don't be ashamed to admit you are on a diet.** If you are conspicuously fat and eating what the other guests are eating, they are probably wondering why you are not on a diet. If you are approaching skinny and dieting because you want to shed those final 10 pounds, or you are maintaining and just eating for optimum nutrition and extra energy, you can get away with anything.

- **Compromise with condition, concede with dignity,** and leave your guilt, along with your fat, behind you. There will almost certainly be times when you're stuck . . . when you can't just "do your own thing" without creating a drama, when you will have to compromise. Just keep in mind that tomorrow is another day. Unlike the past, where tomorrow often meant unfulfilled good intentions and broken diet promises, this is a tomorrow packed with hope and fulfillment. You are in the process of creating an eternal Skinny, so don't let a particular situation or place dictate what you eat. Make your own choices. Stay in control. If you please yourself, you'll end up pleasing the rest of the world, too.

- Check your watch when you arrive at the party and ignore the food for 15 minutes. Once you decide to dig in, don't hover. Deprogram that demonic hand-to-mouth action. Move around— and away from—the food.

- Know that as soon as you put something in your mouth, someone will ask you a question. It's difficult to tell someone your name with a mouthful of meatballs.

- Think about how socially attractive you are when your hands and mouth are loaded with food. It's not easy to give a friend a hug with a glass of wine in one hand and a chicken wing in the other. Tell me, are you likely to seek out the person with the sauce dripping down his or her chin or the conversationalist in the center of the room, far away from the food, whose hands are free to shake yours?

- Beware of nibbling to fill social gaps and of the things you pop in your mouth that don't even taste good. Remember them and record them in your diet diary along with the other foods you've eaten. It will serve as a reminder of what to avoid next time.

- If something doesn't taste good, you don't have to swallow it. Just spit it out—discreetly, of course.

- Keep reminding yourself that this is a social occasion, not simply an eating occasion, and that there will be many more in the future. Try to concentrate on the conversation, not the food. And have fun . . . *you're getting skinny!*

HOLIDAYS

Traditionally, holidays have always represented an opportunity to go crazy. These are special occasions when all of your excuses are allowed, when everybody is blowing it. No one is watching. But that's the old diet consciousness that says holidays are the last supper.

Remember, there is no need for you, as a Born-Again Skinny, to eat yourself under the table because there is nothing on that table you can't have, not if you ate your fruit in the morning and kept yourself "enzymatically open" by avoiding protein and eating only carbohydrates. Remember, once you eat protein, 80 percent of what you eat for the remainder of the day should be protein.

Think of holidays as a testing ground for your new consciousness. This is the time to let your Skinny voice shout. Skinny people don't get crazy just because it is Thanksgiving, Christmas or Easter. They know when enough is enough and so do you. Why not watch a skinny person eat and try to emulate him or her, reminding yourself that *it's not how much you eat in how short a time, it is how long you can make the pleasure last.* Remember, if you don't eat it all today, it will still be here tomorrow.

If you are trying to lose weight and a holiday falls on a specific-food diet day and you want to participate in the eating aspect of the holiday, then go ahead and indulge. Give yourself permission to enjoy the holiday without guilt, but follow the rules for modifying (see "Modifying the Plan," p. 105).

Then, when next Thanksgiving comes, you'll have something more to be thankful for: the body you've always dreamed of and the means to keep it that way forever.

BIRTHDAYS

Your birthday is your day and nobody else's, and that can make it a real let-loose day. Even those who harp about our fat will take us out, pile the food high and urge us on. Well, this year you'll have something to celebrate—being a Born-Again Skinny. You don't have to use your birthday as an excuse anymore . . . you don't need one!

To reinforce my own life choice of being a Skinny, because that 180-pound whale that I once was is always lurking, I choose to make my birthday one of the most austere days of the year. It is almost like a day of worship and reverence for myself, my health and my skinny being.

I know all too well that what once was, could be again. I always know that the fat person can return; that those little fat cells are poised at attention, waiting eagerly for their chance to plump back up. Instead of eating to celebrate my birthday, I buy myself a present. I make it something special that I've looked forward to all year.

However, if instead of following my example, you choose to celebrate with food, that's okay, too. Just give yourself permission and then enjoy. If necessary, just turn to "Corrective Counterparts" (p. 111) and you'll recover. If you are modifying your scheduled weight-loss day, follow the rules for modifying that appear in "Modifying the Plan" (p. 105).

WEDDINGS AND BANQUETS

These deserve a separate category because they have one thing in common: the food is prepared en masse. Think about it: do you really want to blow it on a meal prepared for hundreds? Before I attend such an event, I have my fruit in the morning and eat only carbohydrates prior to the function. That way I'm enzymatically open and prepared for anything.

Since I know that I can only get away with so many open meals, and since most banquet food isn't worth wasting one on, I generally stick to all carbohydrates because the protein portions are usually too small to be satisfying and it's difficult to get more. There's always a salad (you can usually get a second or third), and bread and butter are in abundance. Please, don't be shy about asking for things. It's easy for most public facilities to be accommodating; after all, that's their business. You can even call the catering department ahead of time and ask for a special meal. You'll almost always be able to get baked potatoes or a vegetable plate or, yes, even fruit if you happen to be on a scheduled weight-loss day and you don't want to deviate. If, however, you haven't thought about calling in advance, I repeat, don't be shy. Take a chance and ask on the spot. Most group-oriented facilities will be able to accommodate you without blinking an eye.

Of course, there are always exceptions where you know the food is going to be terrific. In those cases, go ahead and enjoy the occasion, enjoy the food and enjoy the fact that you are developing a technique for eating so that the food won't enjoin you.

RESTAURANTS

Of course you should go out to eat. I don't expect you to be a hermit. As I said earlier, you are not, under any circumstances, allowed to make social sacrifices. This is most important while you are trying to lose weight. I repeat, you cannot build a wall around yourself and expect to adapt my way of eating to your lifestyle, let alone develop your Skinny voice.

Going to a restaurant, however, is not license to go crazy, pig out and blow it. Although we'd like to use the excuse that the exciting, permissible atmosphere of a good restaurant makes it the best exception, it isn't. Consider for a moment the sheer number of restaurants. Then just count the number of times in any given week you are in one. Clearly, each time you visit a restaurant won't be your last, so you've got to stop thinking of them as an exception.

I admit that going to restaurants can be disconcerting while you are on a weight-loss program. It can be particularly difficult at first if frequent restaurant dining is a regular aspect of your lifestyle. Try to stay on track with your eating plan as much as possible. Substituting one carbohydrate for another or one protein for another—eating potatoes instead of corn or a lamb chop instead of chicken—isn't a problem, and neither are occasional deviations or modifications from your all-fruit meals. Remember, however, the enzymes in the fruit are critical to your weight loss, and too many deviations from eating your scheduled fruit will slow down your losing time. Unless the length of time it takes you to lose weight isn't important, it is best to deviate from the fruit meals only if you must.

Now, that doesn't mean that if you are on a grape day and you find yourself in a steak house, you should just sit there drinking black coffee shrouded in martyrdom while everyone around you indulges. You'll be miserable and so will everyone else. Trust me, as long as you are eating something, even if it is only grapes, most people will relax (remember, you can always drink champagne or any kind of wine with fruit).

How do you order grapes in a steak house? You do and you don't. It's easy! Remember you are not the only one on a diet. Restaurants often get special requests, and any good restaurant will make every effort to accommodate you.

Call the restaurant in advance and explain to the maitre d' that you are on a special diet. Tell him what you'll need and ask if he can provide it. (Believe me, it's only hard the first time.) If the restaurant can't provide the food you need, ask if they'll serve you your own food if you bring it with you.

As I said, it's easy, it's fun and it all becomes a game. Don't let restaurants dictate your demise! They don't have to, and you never have to be a victim or a martyr if you always go prepared.

If you can't or haven't called the restaurant in advance, or if it's a casual spot that would make calling ahead uncomfortable, take your food with you and speak to the host or hostess upon arriving. Explain your situation; that this is all you can eat and would they please be kind enough to serve it to you.

Of course, I always offer to pay a service charge of whatever a normal meal would cost. After all, it is presumptuous of us to think we can monopolize a seat in a restaurant without paying. It is the way they make their money. Despite this fact, you probably won't be charged. If there is no maitre d', host or hostess, tell the waiter or waitress what you're up to and then offer to pay. I really doubt that you'll actually have to pay. I never have, nor has anyone I've ever been with.

Since restaurants will always be a part of your life, now is the time to put them into perspective. You can't let them interfere with your skinniness, not if you want to continue to see those same skinny numbers appearing on your scale.

TRAVEL

ON THE ROAD

Just as restaurants are a constant in your life, so is travel. Never forget that *The New Beverly Hills Diet* is a way of life to be integrated into every aspect of your life. You do eat when you travel, don't you? Like restaurants, travel must be integrated into your new skinny ways, not used as an excuse to make exceptions in your choice of foods.

Trips in the car are easy. Just take your food with you. Bagels and dried fruit are my constant traveling companions. Usually the restaurants at your destination are far superior to those en route, but if there are some good stops along the way and you know about them in advance, you should plan to schedule them in. In fact, looking for and stopping at unique local eateries while on motor trips is one of my cherished diversions.

Always remember to make any restaurant stop worth it. Save your diversions for good restaurants and pass up, pass by and pass on the myriad of fast-food establishments you'll see along the way.

IN THE AIR

I know there's not much else to do when you are locked in an airplane except eat, but do you really have to eat *their* food? Since when have TV dinners become your meal of choice? I know it is free and it comes with the ride, but just as there are no free rides, there are no free foods—it always costs you something. If not in dollars and cents, it will cost you those numbers you so love to see on the bathroom scale. And, as I said, if you do eat, do you *really* have to eat *their* food? When you could have your choice of anything in the world, why would you choose airplane food?

Prepared en masse, pre-cooked and heated up for the occasion, airline food can't begin to compare with anything you can have in real life, other than perhaps a high-end diner dinner. First class or coach, it really doesn't matter, and unfortunately it keeps getting worse. On my last cross-country trip I was served an inedible burrito that didn't even compare to a burrito from the lowliest of fast-food stands. When I asked for some bread and butter as a replacement, the stewardess graciously accommodated me. Unfortunately, the butter was not butter; it was one of those disgusting no-butter spreads . . . there wasn't even any real butter on board. Of course, I knew better than to trust fate and bit happily into one of the bagels I'd brought along for the occasion.

Airplane trips, particularly long ones, are great for nibbling, so why not take advantage of them? There are lots of foods you can easily take with you. Just use your imagination and let the time of day and length of the trip determine your choices. In the morning, I usually take fruit or bagels. For flights later in the day, my choices range from nuts to unsalted chips or popcorn. I've even taken cold chicken or a great sandwich I've made at home or purchased on the way. I've yet to peer at my neighbor's tray and not feel infinitely superior for my choice of foods.

If you are still not convinced, or if you are opposed to bringing your own food, then try one of the special-order meals. The salt-free meal is a good choice, as regular meals are inordinately salty. Also, if you order a salt-free meal, at least you won't bloat as a result of retaining all the water you'll need to drink to wash it down. Seafood is also a good choice because it will probably be the tastiest of all the other traditional special-meal choices. Unless it's Hindu or Asian, forget the vegetarian plate; you'll only be disappointed. Despite my undying efforts, despite throwing my weight around (maybe I just don't weigh enough), I've never been successful in ordering and receiving a regular vegetarian meal without cheese, or a salad without either sesame seeds or cheese (hardly worth the miscombination). Besides which, the salads are usually so small they'd barely fill a snail's stomach. And please . . . forgo the fruit plates of apples, oranges and grapefruit accompanied by cottage cheese or yogurt!

Seasoned travelers and Conscious Combiners know that gorging in the air significantly compounds

Believe me, you'll feel much better physically and mentally if you eat your own food, and your body will surely say thank you.

WHEN YOU GET THERE

Travel should not be an occasion to deviate or modify once you get where you are going. Like restaurants, travel has always served as a great excuse to blow it. But you don't need an excuse anymore. What can't you eat? What can't you have? Just follow the basics of Conscious Combining and you can enjoy your vacation—and the food. You don't want to come home and have to put all your new Skinny clothes in storage, do you?

Travel is a good time to test your Skinny voice. If you are on vacation, it may be overly ambitious to expect to stick to the exact 35-day Born-Again Skinny program. . . . A watermelon day while skiing in Aspen? Eating papaya while touring the pyramids in Egypt? Or a dinner of only baked potatoes at a four-star restaurant in Paris? It's not necessary, so don't even try.

You know you can modify or deviate without it being your demise. You have permission! You are creating a lifestyle eating program. You are not on a diet. This isn't only about losing weight. More important, this is about living and enjoying your new life in the slim lane! So eat and enjoy, and as long as you play by the rules, you'll end up a winner, or better yet . . . a loser!

Mind over Matter

Experts tell us that exercise is a major factor in helping us cope with problems by reducing stress and tension as well as controlling our appetite—appetite, I might add, that is more often than not an emotional response to an emotional or stressful situation. We "eaters"—those of us who love to eat and live to eat—are also feelers. Unfortunately, during difficult times we often eat instead of feel. We eat our hearts out. We swallow our anger. We swallow our hurt. We swallow our pride. We swallow our feelings.

If all exercise does for us is allow us to vent our feelings instead of eating, that's certainly nothing to sneer at. Although exercise is vital to mental health and critical to maintaining a healthy heart and good circulation, it is not a compulsory part of this program. Whether you exercise or not, it will have little, if any, effect on your weight loss.

The key to losing weight is not burning calories through exercise, it is eating the correct combinations of foods. Your food choices are what will get you thin and keep you thin. The natural enzymes in the fruit are going to help burn fat and counteract the weight-gaining potential of so-called "fattening" foods.

Slow metabolism is not the culprit. Remember, there is no such thing. You can control your metabolism. You can speed it up by combining foods effectively. You do not have to do anything physical to increase your metabolism; burning calories happens automatically when you practice my technique of Conscious Combining.

Remember, metabolism is the third step of the digestive process. If food is efficiently and sufficiently broken down into nutrients and those nutrients are then absorbed as they should be, they will then metabolize efficiently. The calories resulting from the conversion of the food you've ingested become your body's energy. Food can only make you fat if it has not actually been converted to calories. A calorie becomes a calorie by combustion; you don't have to create the combustion, it is the natural phenomenon of a calorie—that's what makes a calorie a calorie!

This concept is the basis of Conscious Combining, the fundamental principle of *The New Beverly Hills Diet* and my Born-Again Skinny program. True, it flies in the face of everything you've been taught to believe, but if counting calories actually worked, if exercising like a lunatic and eating next to nothing worked, we'd all be thin. Sixty million Americans wouldn't be fat, particularly the millions on a regular exercise regimen. In my opinion, the only reason exercise helps reduce weight is because the person exercising is too busy exercising to eat!

This is not to say that I don't recommend exercise. On the contrary, I couldn't live without my personal routine. I recognize the importance of exercise for the healthful effects it has on our cardiovascular system and mental well-being. I simply don't insist upon it. It has been my experience that when exercise is a requirement of a weight-loss program, we are more apt to lose the dieter than help the dieter lose the weight.

In general, most people with weight to lose are already so riddled with guilt that piling on the added burden and distraction of *having* to exercise is self-defeating. It all becomes too much and before you know it, it is another one of those "I tried it, but I . . ." disappointments. Any change in eating habits, even Conscious Combining, requires discipline. Physical exercise also requires discipline. If you are unsure of your ability to stay focused on your primary task of losing weight, then it is best to forgo exercise for a while. You should take on only one thing at a time.

Now don't get me wrong, I'm not trying to discourage you from exercising. I'm only being conservative and realistic. I've been at this a long time and I know what works. As a rule, "eaters" are most often over-achievers. In our desperate attempt toward self-improvement (as in everything else), we set unrealistic goals for ourselves. These expectations only serve to undermine us. We literally and figuratively bite off more than we can chew, and we choke in the process. So, just start slowly and be realistic in setting your schedule and your goals.

What type of exercise is best for you? Only you can be the judge of that. There are countless organized, disorganized and unorganized physical activities, ranging from a solitary walk to an aerobics class filled with people. Make a list of all the physical activities that tickle your fancy and try each one of them. Then stick to the ones you like best. If, or when, they no longer feel good, it's time to try something else.

If you get bored or you start dreading your chosen activity, don't push yourself. It is time to move on to something else on your list. Nowhere is it written that you must do one exercise forever. If you ease into your exercise routine, you'll make it easy and you'll make it fun. Keep it fun, and you'll enjoy and delight in the new, proud body you are creating.

I know that belonging to a health club is the rage these days, but please don't run right out and join one. You probably won't continue going, and you'll just be wasting your money. If you want to go to an organized class, that's fine. Just don't sign up for any expensive long-term commitments, at least not at first. In the beginning, pay as you go.

For starters, you should engage in a maximum of two classes a week. If you start out with an unrealistic routine—"I'll go every day!"—as is often the case with the born-again exerciser, you are setting yourself up to fail. Your guilt feelings at not being able to keep it up will cause you to give it up. If after one month you want to increase the classes, then by all means do so.

Your best bet to begin exercising is something you can do on your own, something that's easy, convenient and free; then you'll never have to say you can't afford it. If it is something close to your home or your place of business, travel and time can never be used as an excuse.

Walking is a great way to get started, and it doesn't require any athletic prowess. But please don't start with an overly ambitious distance. That infamous "two miles" that is so often mentioned is ridiculous; you'll never keep it up. No, you won't keep up one mile, either. When I say start slow, I mean start slow. For the first three days try one block each way. Then, every three days increase it by a block, until you reach a distance with which you are comfortable. Maintain that distance until you are forced to go farther; until the distance you are doing is simply not enough and you must do more. Ideally, a good exercise program should always leave you a little hungry and wanting more. That way it will always be something you want to do, something you'll look forward to doing, something you'll continue doing.

Experimenting with many different kinds of exercise has given me a wealth of choices, and my exercise of choice is yoga.

Stretch up and you'll feel up. When you stretch your body you stretch yourself, when you reach to infinity, you realize that there is no limit to your potential. No form of exercise aligns your body and mind or gives you more mental and physical strength than yoga. The word yoga actually means union, and practicing it truly does offer the union of body, mind and soul. My body really began to take shape when I changed from the mindless exercises I had been doing to yoga, an exercise that made me think.

Aside from improving my physical well-being and concentration, yoga has enabled me to change my mental attitude. I now strive to accept the challenge of doing, not simply of achieving. When you learn to take control of your body through the development of the improved concentration you'll derive from yoga's focusing techniques, you'll really be able to take control of your life and your eating.

There are many different styles of Hatha yoga (Hatha is the "generic" term encompassing all yoga systems involving body movement). Some are more challenging than others. As a beginner, it isn't necessary to seek out the easiest. The object of yoga, as I said, is not in achieving the goal or in doing it perfectly. Rather, it is to focus 100 percent of your energy and attention into trying.

If you would like to experience yoga, and I strongly recommend you do, your first choice should be a *Yoga College of India.* Hopefully there will be one in your area. Operated and staffed by people personally trained by famed yoga guru to the stars, Bikram Choudhury, these schools offer the most exciting and effective style of yoga available in the Western world. Plus, you'll be in good company. This is the same style touted by Kareem Abdul-Jabbar, Raquel Welch, and the Phoenix Suns, as well as Dan Marino and many of his Dolphin teammates. You can get more information about classes in your area as well as available tapes and books by calling the Beverly Hills headquarters at (310) 854-5800, or by writing them at 8800 Wilshire Boulevard, Beverly Hills, CA 90210.

Hatha yoga planted the seed, but I really began taking control of my life when I started meditating. When I began to turn my attention inward by practicing a very nonphysical form of yoga called *Kriya Yoga.*

You see, for the most part we are only accustomed to looking outside ourselves for fulfillment. We live in a world that conditions us to believe that outer attainments can give us what we really want. Yet again and again, our experiences show us that nothing external, not the act of eating and not even food, no matter what or how much we shove in, can really fulfill the deep longing within us for something more.

Most of the time we find ourselves striving toward that which always seems to be just beyond our reach. We are caught up in the doing rather than the being; in the action, such as eating, rather than the awareness. It is hard for us to picture a state of complete calmness in which thoughts and feelings cease to dance in perpetual motion.

Practicing the science of meditation offers definitive and direct means of stilling the turbulence of your thoughts and the restlessness of your body so that you can begin to know, feel and understand your *Self*.

Since, by nature, our awareness and energy are directed outward, our emotional responses are most often a result of misunderstood external stimuli. It is only when you reverse that flow of energy and consciousness, and turn it inward to your Self, that any real definitive changes in your perception of reality can occur.

This state of perfection, as elusive and impossible as it may seem, this harmony of balance achieved by connecting with your Self, is possible for each one of us. Definitely attainable, it exists within all of us. By meditating on a regular basis, you will uncover that buried perfection within yourself.

Meditating is not something you can learn to do on your own. Contrary to what you may think, meditation isn't just sitting quietly with your eyes closed. It is a science with very definite, easy-to-learn techniques. I highly recommend it for anyone working on reclaiming control of his or her weight and life.

There are many books and classes on meditation, and there is the method that I personally practice. It is this method that I recommend without reservation or hesitation to all of you. It will, no doubt, change your life as it changed mine.

First introduced to the West by Paramahansa Yogananda, author of the critically acclaimed *Autobiography of a Yogi*, the very affordable home-study course of lessons in the technique is available through the nondenominational organization he established in 1925, Self-Realization Fellowship. I urge you to call or write them today at their Los Angeles headquarters: Self-Realization Fellowship, 3880 San Rafael Avenue, Los Angeles, CA 90065, (213) 225-2471.

And now it's time to get thin. . . . Forever!

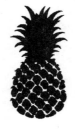

PART II

Born-Again Skinny

Anchors Aweigh

Enough said . . . well, almost. There are a few last-minute instructions before you actually begin. Don't worry if you don't understand all the "why's" and "wherefore's"—I don't expect you to. I guarantee you'll understand it all as the days unfold and all your questions are answered!

If you turn to p. 98, you'll find a place to put your "before" picture. Now, don't just find a recent picture, take a new one. Believe me, this, like everything else I ask you to do, is crucial to your success. Also, please make sure you take your picture before you actually begin the program, not after you've already started. You'll realize the importance of this picture as you move through the program. It will become a constant source of inspiration.

Following your "before" picture page is your "after" picture page, the picture you are going to take five weeks from now. This will be the new you, the you that you've always wanted to be and are about to become!

I've left a few blank pages at the end of the diary in the event that you haven't lost all your weight in the 35 days. (Again, 15 pounds is the average.) Don't worry, once you've completed your 35 days there will be instructions on how to keep going if you still have more weight to lose. You should take and add a new picture every 35 days until you reach your goal. And you will reach your goal; I'll see to that!

Now, let's get into the meat—or should I say the bare bones—of the diet: the food you are going to eat.

If you turn to the "Diet List" (p. 107), you'll find the 35 days of the diet listed in consecutive order. That's so you can be prepared for each day and shop in advance. You shouldn't have a problem finding any of the fruits. The success of my first book—and the millions of people still following my original program— has virtually made papayas and mangoes as readily available as bananas. In the event your local grocer doesn't carry them, he can easily order them. In addition to the full listing, there is also a "Mini Daily Diary" (pp. 120-121). This is where each individual day, complete with the food you'll be eating, is shown in its own box. I've left a little space for you to make some notes and to add some pertinent information. Although the days of the week are already noted, I've left blank spaces for you to fill in the dates.

As you can see, Day 1 is a Monday; that's because I want you to start on a Monday. Actually, I don't just *want* you to start on a Monday, I *insist* that you do. You'll see, I have my reasons.

In the upper right-hand corner of each day you'll find a space to record your weight. That's right: *every single day,* come what may, even if you've been naughty and cheated ("cheating" is a word that you will soon drop from your vocabulary soon . . . at least as far as your diet is concerned), you are going to weigh yourself. First thing every morning I want you to jump on that scale—preferably naked or at least almost naked—and write those numbers in your book. Don't eat or drink anything before you weigh in. That way, we will get your most accurate weight, the one by which we will measure your progress.

I know that for many of you stepping onto that scale is going to be *very* difficult. You won't believe some of the excuses I've heard people use for not weighing themselves. The one I like the best is, "Oh, I didn't have time . . ." Like three seconds is a long time? But no matter how much you hate it now, before you know it, that "iron monster"—your scale— will become your best friend.

If you don't have a scale, you must go out and get one immediately because you cannot begin the diet until you do. It doesn't have to be expensive. My personal preference is a non-digital type. If it is not 100 percent accurate, that's okay, as long as it is consistent. If it is a pound light or heavy, that is not important. What is important is the movement; its downward trend, I mean!

Now turn back to the "Diet List" (p. 107) so we can talk a little bit about the diet itself. You'll notice that the foods are listed in a very specific order. This order lists them in the sequence in which they are to be eaten. Don't switch them around or skip any. If a specific amount is listed, you must eat that amount. When I say eight ounces, I mean eight ounces. Not six, not four, but eight! It doesn't have to be in one sitting. Remember, this is not a three-meal-a-day plan. You aren't confined to breakfast, lunch and dinner. You may stop and start as you wish, but do not go on to the next food listed until you have finished the required amount of the first.

As I said in the introduction, you are going to lose weight by feeding your body, not by starving it. If a food is listed and an amount is not shown, then you can eat as much of that food as you want. There are no restrictions. With fruit, in particular, the more you eat the more you'll lose. So eat a lot. You have permission to really get full.

Now don't get me wrong. I'm not telling you to stuff yourself. I just don't want you to go hungry. I repeat, you are not confined to the traditional breakfast, lunch and dinner regimen. You can eat as often as you want. You can eat whenever you feel hungry—as long as you follow the plan.

It is very important that you eat fresh fruit and vegetables. Frozen and canned foods are only acceptable when fresh is not available and you've exhausted all avenues for finding them.

Fresh fruit, however, is not, I repeat, not a substitute for dried fruit. This is important. You need the concentrated nutrition that you'll be getting from the dried fruits I have instructed you to eat. And again, please try to make sure the dried fruits do not contain sulfur dioxide and potassium sorbate. Read the labels carefully. You'll probably have to purchase these in a health food store or a large grocery store with a health food section. I hope you have one in your area. Remember, you are feeding your body and eliminating the toxic residues stored in your fat deposits. Adding more chemicals will just inhibit the process, so try your hardest to find the right foods.

If you can't find unsulfured dried fruits in your area, write or call my ClubSlim headquarters, or visit *The New Beverly Hills Diet* World Wide Web site, and we'll tell you how you can receive them by mail. The contact information is listed at the end of the book.

Now, it's true that you aren't counting fat grams; however, **how** the oil you consume has been processed is very important. You want it to be **unrefined** or **cold-pressed,** so check the label for those words. You should be able to find these oils in the health food section of your regular market and certainly at any specialty health food store, or they can be ordered through ClubSlim.

You can drink all the water, coffee and tea (hot or iced) that you want, but no milk, non-dairy creamers or artificial sweeteners. Sugar is all right, but use it only if you must. I know you are saying, "But sugar is so bad for you." Chemical food additives, my friend, are much worse!

If you find that you can't drink your coffee black, please don't give up the coffee; you'll probably miss it too much. But don't try sneaking the milk in, either. Milk is a protein and it will inhibit your weight loss. (Remember the protein rule! See chapter 5.) There are some very fine rice- and soy-milk products available in most markets. A product called Rice Dream is the one many people prefer.

Real butter, preferably unsalted, is not only okay, it is **all** you can use. Unless your doctor has insisted upon it, you are absolutely not permitted margarine or, heaven forbid, that "no-butter" butter or lite-butter junk.

One more "no." **No diet sodas,** and, like the milk, don't try to sneak them in either, not if you want to lose weight. They are loaded with sodium and chemicals. If giving them up will drive you crazy, an occasional real soda is allowed. But when I say "occasional," I mean not more than one every two to three days. And don't fudge, don't try to slip in extras; you'll only hurt yourself.

Midnight does not a new day make. The day ends when you go to sleep at night; and the new day begins when you wake up in the morning. If you awaken hungry in the middle of the night, eat more of the last thing you ate before you went to sleep.

THE DAILY DIARY

Now, let's talk about the diary itself. You'll notice that it is divided into daily chapters in "Born-Again Skinny Day by Day." Each chapter should be read in order, one day at a time. Starting your day with the diary's boost of support is very important, so try to read it first thing in the morning, not just at some point during the day. Reading it just before going to sleep the night before is also a good idea.

Reading your daily diary chapter shouldn't take you more than 10 minutes. The support and information provided in those 10 minutes, however, are crucial to your ultimate success as you'll not only get your lesson in my technique, but I will also give you tips and pointers on the foods you'll be eating. Equally, if not more important, will be the soul food I will provide, the nourishment that's going to inspire and encourage you to stick to your diet—and change your way of thinking. Remember, my program is as much a philosophy (a way of thinking) as it is a methodology (a way of eating).

So, read your diary chapters first thing each morning, and just as you wouldn't skip around in a novel or read the ending first, don't read the days ahead of themselves. Stop at the end of each day—this is vital to your success. Trust me, I want this to work for you—and it will. Believe me, I know what's best for you. It has taken me years to develop this program. My teachings have been tried and tested, and I know just how much of it you can digest at a time. I only want you to become thin, and you will . . . if you do it my way.

Of course, you can reread your daily chapters as often as you'd like. In fact, I encourage the repetition. This also applies to any of the other diary chapters you've already read. They are filled with a wealth of information and inspiration, not all of which you'll catch the first time around.

The diary is your ticket to the world of eternal slimhood.

Okay, now it really is time to begin.

I want you to stand in front of a full-length mirror, or one that shows as much of your body as possible. Take your book with you, you'll need it. Are you there? Okay, now put your hands on your hipbones, or where you think your hipbones might be. For those of you who can't see or feel them yet, trust me—you will soon.

Now repeat after me . . .

"I used to be fat. I'm not fat anymore, and I'll NEVER be fat again!"

Good luck, Skinny! I know you are going to be my best example!

The
Born-Again Skinny
Diary

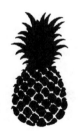

BEFORE PICTURE

The Fat I Soon Won't Be!

AFTER PICTURE

The New Skinny Me!

What I Hate About Being Fat

1. _____
2. _____
3. _____
4. _____
5. _____
6. _____
7. _____
8. _____
9. _____
10. _____

What's So Great About Being Thin?

1. _____
2. _____
3. _____
4. _____
5. _____
6. _____
7. _____
8. _____
9. _____
10. _____

Rehash Sheet

_____

_____

_____

_____

_____

_____

_____

_____

_____

_____

_____

_____

_____

_____

_____

Mind-over-Matter Rules

1. Think about food when it doesn't count, so you don't have to think about food when it does.
2. Make every bite count—for every bite that goes into your mouth, something else cannot.
3. What you choose to eat determines what you have to eat.
4. It is not how much you can eat in how short a time, but how long you can make the pleasure last.
5. If you don't have it now, you can have it later. If you don't have it later, you can have it tomorrow. **Nothing is leaving the planet.**

Golden Rules

1 Weigh yourself *every* day, no matter what.

2 **Fruit.** Start almost every day of your life with fruit. Once you have gone off fruit in the course of the day, never, never ever go back to it.

Remember, fruit digests almost instantly. Before you can even finish eating a pineapple, its nutrients are being absorbed by your body. If it is inhibited in its digestion, if it is eaten after anything else, it gets trapped in your stomach by other foods. Its explosive enzyme action will be offset by bloating and gas. Your savior will be transformed into your torment.

3 **The waiting time.** When you go from fruit to fruit, wait one hour. When you go from one food group to another, wait two hours minimum (three would be better).

These are the minimum waiting times—the shortest periods of time you can get away with without running the risk of fat. Remember, you gain weight because food is not processed properly. In simpler terms, if food doesn't leave your stomach when it should, if it becomes trapped or held up by other antagonistic foods, the nutrients it should generate will not be properly processed by your body and you'll gain weight.

4 **Protein.** Once you've eaten protein, eat at least 80 percent protein for the remainder of the day.

Modifying the Plan

Critical to achieving maximum weight loss is following the program exactly. You can expect a 10- to 15-pound loss in the 35 days. Unlike a typical "diet," this program takes the weight off not by starving your body, but by feeding it. Food and eating are what will make you thin and keep you thin. Eating the specific foods in the order listed is vital, so please do not deviate. There are some allowable substitutions listed in the "Substitute Food List" (p. 109) just in case you're allergic to a specific food or there's something on the diet you really hate. However, because each food has a definite purpose, substitute only if you must.

If you have just a few pounds to lose or are simply trying to maintain your weight, you may want to modify the program. It's easy: simply begin your day with the scheduled food, eat enough so that you are really full, wait two hours and then eat whatever you would normally eat. That doesn't meant "pig out" or go crazy; likewise, don't starve yourself either. If you want to do two-thirds of the day my way and then do your own thing, that's also fine. Even throwing in an occasional whole day my way is great, too. Just follow the program in the right daily order. Of course, you'll lose the most weight the fastest if you follow the diet to the letter.

Even if you are modifying the plan, it is important to weigh yourself every day and read your daily chapter because it will further explain my technique and how to apply it to your lifestyle and your favorite foods. You'll see, it won't be long before you'll find that doing things my way—Conscious Combining— will become your way as well.

If you have a lot of weight to lose, you can still follow the modified plan, but I don't recommend it. These initial 35 days will be the best thing that ever happened to you. You may think you can't do it, but you can. Then again, you are the best judge of you. So if you must modify, then modify. It is better than doing nothing at all.

Now give me your hand, you little Skinny, and I'll lead you out of the Valley of the Shadow of Fat, and together we'll revel in the Land of Hipbones.

Diet List

DAY 1 Pineapple; corn on the cob and LTO salad with Mazel dressing*

DAY 2 Prunes (8 oz.); strawberries; baked potatoes

DAY 3 Grapes

DAY 4 Dried apricots (8 oz.); mini Mazel salad;* pasta

DAY 5 Pineapple; papaya; pineapple

DAY 6 Papaya; steak or lamb chops, and shrimp, any style

DAY 7 Pineapple; Mazel salad*

DAY 8 Grapes; (raisins/popcorn optional)

DAY 9 Prunes (8 oz.); strawberries; chicken or turkey

DAY 10 Dried apricots (8 oz.); papaya; pineapple

DAY 11 Watermelon

DAY 12 Dried apricots (8 oz.); avocado sandwich; 3 vegetables of choice with rice

DAY 13 Grapes; 2 bananas

DAY 14 Pineapple; strawberries; open with discretion**

DAY 15 Pineapple; Mazel salad*

DAY 16   Dried apricots (8 oz.); papaya; pineapple

DAY 17   Watermelon

DAY 18   Figs; dessert of choice; meat/protein

DAY 19   Mango or papaya; pineapple; artichokes, asparagus
or potatoes, any style

DAY 20   Kiwi; open with discretion;** protein

DAY 21   Pineapple; 2 bananas

DAY 22   Grapes or cherries; bedtime treat

DAY 23   Prunes (8 oz.); sandwich of choice; fisherman's
platter/protein

DAY 24   Pineapple; papaya; pineapple

DAY 25   Watermelon

DAY 26   On your own***

DAY 27   On your own***

DAY 28   Pineapple; papaya; pineapple

DAY 29   Watermelon or grapes

DAY 30   Prunes (8 oz.); vegetable sandwich; vegetable ethnic/open
carbohydrate

DAY 31   Orange juice and choice of honeydew, cantaloupe or
$1/2$ grapefruit; sandwich of choice; protein

DAY 32   Protein

DAY 33   Pineapple; 2 bananas

DAY 34   Pineapple; papaya; pineapple

DAY 35   Watermelon or grapes

---

* Recipes appear on pp. 131, 148-150 and 162.

** "Open with discretion" will be fully explained on Day 14. DO NOT
READ AHEAD. Wait—you'll be pleasantly surprised.

*** Wait until Day 26 to find out what "On your own" means. Trust
me, you'll have fun.

Substitute Food List

Fruit on Program	Substitute Fruit
Strawberries	Pineapple, kiwi
Kiwi	Mango, papaya, persimmon, or apples (a last resort)
Figs or dates	Prunes, raisins
Papaya	Mango, kiwi, persimmon
Mango	Papaya, kiwi, persimmon
Pineapple	Strawberries
Prunes	Figs
Watermelon*	8 oz. dried apricots (morning) Pineapple (midday) Fresh asparagus (evening)
Grapes*	6 oz. prunes (morning) Strawberries, blueberries or raisins (midday) 8 oz. raw Brazil nuts (evening)

* The substitutes are no comparison to the real thing. Substitute for watermelon or grapes only if you must.

Drastic Measures
After a Drastic Disaster

You lost control, broke your diet, ate everything in sight . . .

If you are up *any* less than five pounds, you simply eat fruit for two-thirds of the day (see "Corrective Counterparts," pp. 111-112) and a properly combined meal at night. The meal should be either all protein or all carbohydrates, your choice. Or, choose either diet Day 1, 2, 6 or 14. Do that day, then resume the diet where you left off.

If your weight is up **five pounds or more**, follow these recoup days for one to four days in precise order, but never more than once per month.

Day 1.   Pineapple; papaya; pineapple

Day 2.   Watermelon

Day 3.   Prunes; strawberries; baked potatoes, cooked spinach with oil

Day 4.   Grapes

You should never need more than four days to recoup from the worst of eating indiscretions.

Corrective Counterparts

Antidotes and precedotes are used to offset the negative side effects of eating foods that are difficult to digest. Precedotes are foods eaten for breakfast the day you know you'll be eating the types of foods listed. Antidotes are foods eaten for breakfast the day following the indiscretion.

Before You Eat	Precedote
Greasy, creamy, cheesy	Pineapple or strawberries
Salty	Dried apricots

After You Eat	Antidote
Greasy, creamy, cheesy	Burn with pineapple or strawberries
Protein	Soften and digest with papaya or mango (mango is better after fowl, papaya after meat)

After You Eat	Antidote (cont.)
Sweets	Scrub with grapes
Salty	Wash with watermelon or mop with meat*

* This is very individual. Only you and your scale will know which works best for you. If watermelon doesn't work the first time you experience excessive bloating after a salty meal (that is, if it doesn't make that scale go back down the next day), then make the next day an all-protein day. That should do the trick. If you bloat again after a salty meal, you'll know protein is your antidote.

Food Groups

Proteins

Beef	Kefir	Pork	Desserts:
Cheese	Lamb	Seafood	Cheesecake
Eggs	Milk	Seeds	Crème brûlée
Fish	Nuts	Yogurt	Crème caramel
Fowl	Nut butters		Flan
			Ice cream

Fats

Butter	Mayonnaise	Sour cream
Heavy cream	Oil	Whipped cream

Carbohydrates

Fruits	Mini-Carbohydrates	Midi-Carbohydrates	Maxi-Carbohydrates
(a carb in a category all it's own)	Asparagus	Beets	Artichokes
All fruits	Celery	Broccoli	Barley
Brandy	Crookneck squash	Brussels sprouts	Breads
Champagne	Herbs	Cabbage	Buckwheat
Cognac	Kale	Carrots	Bulgur
Wine	Lettuce	Cauliflower	Cake (white,
	Mushrooms	Cucumbers	sponge, choc-
	Mustard greens	Eggplant	olate, carrot)
	Parsley	Leeks	Chocolate
50/50—	Zucchini	Onions	Cookies
Either/Or		Parsnips	Corn
Avocados		Peas	Cornmeal
Garbanzo beans		Peppers (red,	Couscous
Kidney beans		green and chile)	Cream of Wheat
Lentils		Radishes	Farina
Lima beans		Shallots	Grains
Peanuts		String beans	Millet
Pinto beans		Tomatoes	Oatmeal
Soybeans		Turnips	Oats
			Pasta
			Pie crust
			Potatoes
			Rice
			Rye
			Wheat
			Winter Squash

Alcohol:
  Beer
  All distilled:
    Bourbon, Rum,
    Scotch, Tequila,
    Vodka, etc.

Playing It Straight

Here are a few examples of perfectly combined meals to whet your appetite. Use your imagination and add to these.

All Protein Meals

Bacon, eggs and sausage

Hamburger and eggs

Steak and eggs

Chicken liver omelet

Deli meat platter

Deli platter (scoops of chicken salad, tuna salad, egg salad, chopped liver, white fish salad, etc.)

Shrimp cocktail, lobster, butter

Carpaccio, veal chops, cheesecake

Surf and turf (steak and lobster)

Oysters, lamb chops, ice cream

Fried calamari, Italian sausage, tiramisu

All Carbohydrate Meals

Bagels, tomato, onion, sour cream

Lettuce, tomato and onion sandwich with French fries

Salsa, chips, beer

Onion soup (no cheese), French bread, salad

Vegetable tempura, rice, suinomo salad

Vegetables and baked potato

Avocado, tomato and onion sandwich

Corn on the cob, baked potato and salad

Pasta with tomato and basil, garlic bread and amaretto cookie

Supplements

I have never been a proponent of dietary supplements, but there are a few I consider important.

BRAN

Eat two tablespoons of unprocessed bran flakes first thing in the morning mixed with a small amount of a hot beverage; water is the best. Wait at least 20 minutes before eating anything else. Bran is the ultimate intestinal broom, but it will only sweep effectively on an empty stomach. If it gets clogged up behind other foods, you'll likely bloat.

NUTRITIONAL YEAST (BREWER'S YEAST)

Antibiotics, coffee, chocolate or anything containing caffeine, as well as emotional stress, deplete your body's supply of B vitamins. There is no more effective way of replenishing them than with nutritional yeast. At 4:00 P.M. each day, eat one to two heaping tablespoons of nutritional yeast flakes mixed with a small amount of water to the consistency of peanut butter. Do not eat for 30 minutes before or after eating the yeast. The two brands most highly recommended for their flavor are Kal and Red Star.

SESAME SEEDS

Sesame seeds are the richest natural digestible calcium source available on the planet. All that concentrated calcium will not only be good for your bones (particularly important to women for the prevention of osteoporosis), but it will also help you sleep by relaxing your nervous system. Sesame seeds also provide extra fiber as well as lecithin and the three essential fatty acids you can acquire only from food. At bedtime, eat two heaping tablespoons of raw, unhulled sesame seeds.

An additional calcium supplement is advisable for women. Your doctor would be your best guide in choosing one.

VITAMINS

I also recommend 1,000 mg of a natural vitamin C with bioflavonoids daily, as well as a high-grade natural one-a-day multivitamin. If you feel the need, you can also add a one-a-day multi-mineral supplement to your daily plan.

BLUE-GREEN ALGAE

Although similar products, such as Spirulena and Cholorella, are available, I don't believe they compare to the nutritional wallop packed by Blue-Green Algae. Naturally harvested from a lake in Oregon and freeze-dried, I'm firmly convinced that these little

seaweed tablets are so chock-full of natural nutrients they could actually sustain life if more conven-
tional food were not available. Unfortunately, this
product is not available in retail stores. I'll be happy
to put you in touch with the source if you drop me a
line at my ClubSlim headquarters or at my World
Wide Web site. Contact information is listed in the
back of this book.

For additional nutritional supplement recommen-
dations, ask your doctor.

MINI DAILY DIARY

	MONDAY	TUESDAY	WEDNESDAY
WEEK 1	**Day 1** Date: _____ Wt. _____ Pineapple; corn on the cob, LTO salad w/Mazel dressing	**Day 2** Date: _____ Wt. _____ Prunes (8 oz.); strawberries; baked potatoes	**Day 3** Date: _____ Wt. _____ Grapes
WEEK 2	**Day 8** Date: _____ Wt. _____ Grapes; (raisins or popcorn optional)	**Day 9** Date: _____ Wt. _____ Prunes (8 oz.); strawberries; chicken or turkey	**Day 10** Date: _____ Wt. _____ Dried apricots (8 oz.); papaya; pineapple
WEEK 3	**Day 15** Date: _____ Wt. _____ Pineapple; Mazel salad	**Day 16** Date: _____ Wt. _____ Dried apricots (8 oz.); papaya; pineapple	**Day 17** Date: _____ Wt. _____ Watermelon
WEEK 4	**Day 22** Date: _____ Wt. _____ Grapes or cherries; bedtime treat	**Day 23** Date: _____ Wt. _____ Prunes (8 oz.); sandwich of choice; fisherman's platter/protein	**Day 24** Date: _____ Wt. _____ Pineapple; papaya; pineapple
WEEK 5	**Day 29** Date: _____ Wt. _____ Watermelon or grapes	**Day 30** Date: _____ Wt. _____ Prunes (8 oz.); vegetable sandwich; vegetable ethnic/open carbohydrate	**Day 31** Date: _____ Wt. _____ Orange juice, choice of honeydew, cantaloupe or 1/2 grapefruit; sandwich of choice; protein

THURSDAY	FRIDAY	SATURDAY	SUNDAY
Day 4	**Day 5**	**Day 6**	**Day 7**
Date: _____ Wt. _____ Dried apricots (8 oz.); mini Mazel salad; pasta	Date: _____ Wt. _____ Pineapple; papaya; pineapple	Date: _____ Wt. _____ Papaya; steak or lamb chop, and shrimp, any style	Date: _____ Wt. _____ Pineapple; Mazel salad
Day 11	**Day 12**	**Day 13**	**Day 14**
Date: _____ Wt. _____ Watermelon	Date: _____ Wt. _____ Dried apricots (8 oz.); avocado sandwich; 3 veggies with rice	Date: _____ Wt. _____ Grapes; 2 bananas	Date: _____ Wt. _____ Pineapple; strawberries; open with discretion
Day 18	**Day 19**	**Day 20**	**Day 21**
Date: _____ Wt. _____ Figs; dessert of choice; meat/protein	Date: _____ Wt. _____ Mango or papaya; pineapple; artichokes, asparagus or potatoes, any style	Date: _____ Wt. _____ Kiwi; open with discretion; protein	Date: _____ Wt. _____ Pineapple; 2 bananas
Day 25	**Day 26**	**Day 27**	**Day 28**
Date: _____ Wt. _____ Watermelon	Date: _____ Wt. _____ On your own	Date: _____ Wt. _____ On your own	Date: _____ Wt. _____ Pineapple; papaya; pineapple
Day 32	**Day 33**	**Day 34**	**Day 35**
Date: _____ Wt. _____ Protein	Date: _____ Wt. _____ Pineapple; 2 bananas	Date: _____ Wt. _____ Pineapple; papaya; pineapple	Date: _____ Wt. _____ Watermelon or grapes

Born-Again Skinny

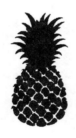

Day by Day

DAY 1

Pineapple
Corn on the Cob
LTO Salad with Mazel Dressing

Well, you did it. You've actually started. It's your first day and, oh boy, what a first day. Corn on the cob for dinner . . . who ever heard of having corn on the cob on a diet, let alone the first day of a diet? I told you it was going to be fun.

Before we go any further, let's talk about salt. Butter on your corn is just fine, but it must be unsalted. And please, no salt on the corn, or the water in which you're boiling it. I know you love salt. Don't worry, you won't have to avoid it forever. Right now, however, you need to be as salt-free as possible to accelerate your weight loss. The high levels of potassium in all the fruits you'll be eating over the next weeks will also help counteract the excess water you're retaining—a hangover from your earlier salt intake.

How much can you eat? How many ears of corn? How much butter? Let your conscience be your guide. If you find yourself going overboard and eating too much, remind yourself why you're doing this. You're trying to lose weight, not beat the system. Trust me, we all have the same problem. You are not alone. All of us "eaters" do the same thing: we try to see how much we can get away with—myself included! That's why I created this program. I wanted to get away with murder, but I didn't want to serve a life sentence. I didn't want to be fat anymore. I've succeeded and so will you.

Back to the amounts . . . most people eat two or three ears of corn, with a couple of pats of butter (about a tablespoon in total). If you miss the salty taste and want to add a little zing, sprinkle on some cayenne or black pepper. That will pep it up. And don't forget to chew. A lot of people complain that they have difficulty digesting corn, but that's only because they don't chew it. As I explained earlier, chewing is very important. For one thing, your stomach doesn't have teeth, so if food isn't sufficiently broken down before it hits your stomach, it is going to slow down the digestive process, causing inefficient digestion—something we want to avoid at all costs. Remember, inefficient digestion is one of the main reasons you are now overweight.

The other reason chewing well is important is that the primary carbohydrate-digesting enzyme, ptyalin, is activated in your saliva when you chew. So if you don't chew, you won't activate the enzyme, and the carbohydrate (that corn on the cob, the baked potatoes with butter you're going to have tomorrow night, the stir-fry vegetables and rice that are just a few days away) will not be digested properly.

Remember, an enzyme is a biological catalyst that turns food into nutrients or, as they are technically called, amino acids, glucose and lipids.

Along with your corn this evening is an LTO salad with Mazel dressing. You'll find the recipes for both at the end of today's diary entry. This salad, simple as it may seem, is my personal favorite. I love the taste and I always feel great after I eat one. It's important to use iceberg lettuce, as called for in the recipe. It, like all the other foods I instruct you to eat, is there for a reason, be it for emotional reasons (you know, those fun foods that we eat to feel good emotionally) or for nutritional reasons (for making your body feel good). In this case, it's for nutritional reasons. We're feeding your body with the very special mineral balance created by the combination in my LTO salad.

You can eat as much salad as you want. The salad is also a carbohydrate, so don't forget to chew and don't gobble. If you find you are eating too fast, just keep reminding yourself that it's not how much you eat in how short a time, it's how long you can make the pleasure last.

I'm not concerned with how much oil you use as long as it is unrefined or cold-pressed. If you're using olive oil, it should be virgin olive oil. If you use good oil it can be healthful and slimming; if you don't, then it will be harmful and fattening.

Now that we've covered dinner, let's talk about the earlier part of the day. Remember how adamant I was that you start with this diet on a Monday? Well, that's because you've always started a diet on a Monday. I believe Fats Domino called it "Blue Monday." Well, today is Monday and you are starting a diet, but it's not just another diet and it is certainly not a Blue

Monday. It is a Sunny Monday, a Monday filled with hope and promise, the promise of eternal slimhood because at last you have found the answer, your cure for fat. With my help you are going to get thin and stay thin, and never again will you have to start your week with another diet. I promise you, do as I say and this is the last diet you will ever have to go on.

Appropriately, you'll begin the program with the fruit that has become synonymous with *The Beverly Hills Diet*, the golden pineapple—my trademark—sweet and luscious, with all its powerful fat-burning enzymes. From the time you begin eating today until two hours before dinner, I want you to eat pineapple, lots and lots of pineapple.

Since this is not a three-meal-a-day program, you are not confined to breakfast, lunch and dinner. With your pineapple, as with all the fruit you'll be eating over the next weeks where no amount is specified, you are to eat as much of it as you want, as often as you can. The more you eat, the more you lose. Your fruit is the catalyst that is accelerating your weight loss.

Now don't get me wrong, I don't want you to stuff yourself, but I want you to feel full. (I do not want to hear, "I'm hungry . . .") There's no reason for you to be hungry; bored maybe, but not hungry. So eat, eat and eat some more!!!

How much pineapple should you eat today? At least one to two whole ones. But you can have more if you desire. Just keep nibbling. But don't forget that you have to wait two hours from the last bite of pineapple to your first bite of corn and salad. Remember the waiting rule of two hours from food group to food group. You may want to review the rules before you start. In fact, I would suggest doing this periodically until you have them committed to memory.

So plan accordingly and be sure to stop eating your pineapple at least two hours before you begin your dinner. The waiting time is critical to the success of this program, so don't stint, not even by five minutes, not if you really want this program to work. You'll see, the pounds are going to fall off. And, when this waiting rule becomes as important to you as the other rules that guide your life, those pounds will stay off forever.

Speaking of pounds, you did weigh yourself today, didn't you? Well, if you didn't, you better get on the scale right now. I can't emphasize strongly enough how important this is. And be sure to write your weight in the appropriate place in your diet diary. After you do, there is one final thing I want you to do: I want you to say your weight aloud. Telling another person is best, but saying it into thin air, out of earshot of anyone, is fine, too. Make this a daily practice. Trust me, there is more to losing weight than just going on a diet. You become a thin person by becoming a thin person, by confronting, acknowledging and letting go of the fat person. You confront your weight by weighing yourself, you acknowledge it by writing it down, and you let go of it when you say it aloud. I know this sounds silly, but it's true. The people who have gone on my program and refused to weigh themselves lost much less weight than those who did, and they invariably gained back whatever they lost.

But you can be certain that's not going to happen to you because I won't let it. This time, you're not only going to lose weight, you are finally going to reach your goal, your ideal weight, whatever that may be. And it won't be determined by any chart or statistics, and it certainly won't be determined by me. Only you know what you want to look like and what numbers you want to see on the scale that say, "You're perfect."

Perfect, by the way, doesn't necessarily mean ultra-thin. It's what you consider right for you. It's when you can honestly say, "I don't have to lose one more pound and I really feel good about that and myself." I don't want you to get on the scale and say, "if only" or "but." I'm not going to let you stop the losing process as long as you are still saying, "Well, I'm okay, but I would be better if . . . ," or "I really need to lose five more pounds," or "I look great but I'd look better two pounds lighter."

Achieving perfection, being able to step on that scale and say "terrific" with no "if only" or "but," is what is going to keep you from gaining back your weight. The satisfaction you'll experience from achieving this state will insure that you'll never get fat again.

This state of perfection may come soon for some, while for others it may seem an eternity away. But regardless of how much you have to lose or how far away you are from your goal, this time you are going to reach it because I'm going to help you. I'm here for you no matter how long it takes. And just think, by the end of today, you'll be a day closer to that goal. Tomorrow your scale will confirm it. If you follow today's program, you'll probably weigh less tomorrow than you did today.

So be good and just remember . . .
    I'm counting on you to be my best example.

LTO Salad

1 large, firm head
  iceberg lettuce
4 tomatoes
1 large red or Spanish
  onion, peeled

1–2 cucumbers, peeled
Mazel dressing or olive oil

With a sharp knife, cut all vegetables into good-sized chunks. Toss with dressing or oil.

YIELD: 2 servings

Mazel Dressing

¼ cup rice vinegar
1 cup sesame oil
Chopped garlic,* to taste
  (1–2 small cloves)

Chopped or grated ginger,*
  to taste
Freshly ground pepper

Combine all ingredients.

YIELD: 1¼ cups

---

* From clove to clove and root to root, garlic and ginger may differ in intensity. If they are left to steep in dressing, their flavors will intensify. Therefore, depending on when you make the dressing, on the strength of the garlic and ginger, and, of course, on personal taste, the amounts used may differ. Start with 1 clove of garlic and 6 or 7 gratings of ginger and increase to three times that amount if desired.

D A Y 2

Prunes
Strawberries
Baked Potatoes

I don't understand why prunes have such a bad reputation. People always snicker at the mere mention of them. It's ridiculous. Not only are they just plain delicious, they also have an enormous amount of nutritional value. In fact, there are very few foods that will provide your body with as much iron and potassium.

Iron is the mineral that helps build red blood cells and triggers enzymes needed by your bones, brain and muscles. Among other things, potassium regulates the electrolyte balance in your cells so that you don't retain excess fluid and bloat; as well as keeping your heart healthy.

You can eat prunes with or without pits, although you'll get more prunes for your eight ounces if they are pitted. Just make sure sulfur dioxide or potassium sorbate has not been added—you'll need to read the contents on the label carefully. If you've purchased them in a health food store, the bag they come in will most probably state "No Sulfur Dioxide Added" in big bold letters.

Speaking of preservatives, let's examine the American diet. Although it exists, you don't see obesity in Europe the way you see it in the United States. In fact, most of my international clientele are constantly complaining about how much weight they gain when they come to this country, despite not changing their eating habits. That's because the foods in the American diet are overloaded with preservatives and chemicals. There is no question in my mind that preservatives and chemicals are partially responsible for the fact that 80 percent of the American population is overweight. Most preservatives are sodium-based. This adds extra, unneeded salt to our bodies, which results in water retention and extra pounds. Also, preservatives cannot be turned into nutrients—the only thing our bodies can properly digest—and anything that can't be properly digested is going to make you fat.

You'll find that eight ounces of prunes are a lot of prunes, far too many to finish in one sitting. They are very rich and chewy, so if you want to discover their magic taste, don't just gobble them down, savor them. You can eat them as they are, straight from the bag, or you can simmer them slowly in water. If you do cook them, drink the water in which they've been cooked. If they seem a bit too dry and are hard to chew, cover them with warm water and soak them for 30 to 60 minutes. Again, drink that water to take full advantage of the nutritional value.

As I said, I don't expect you to eat all eight ounces of prunes in one sitting; you can stop and start eating them as often as you'd like, wherever you'd like, even in your car on the way to work.

I told you there would be no behavior modification. I will never insist that you sit at the table and eat. In fact, the table happens to be my least favorite place to eat. I love to eat while I'm driving, while I'm in the kitchen standing at the counter, in bed or at my desk while I'm talking on the telephone—anywhere but at a table. I could never follow any kind of an eating program that placed that kind of a restriction on me. Since I love to nibble, today's eating program (like most of the days on this program) is heaven for nibblers.

Remember, don't start eating your strawberries until you have finished every last prune and you have taken a one-hour break. As always, be sure to observe the Waiting Rule: When you go from one fruit to another, remember to wait one hour.

When I'm on a prune and strawberry day (and believe me, I didn't go from 180 pounds to 108 pounds without prune and strawberry days), I eat at least three baskets of strawberries. I even leave on some of the green tops. They contain chlorophyll, which helps absorb the fat that the enzymes in the strawberries are burning up.

The enzyme in strawberries, by the way, is *bromelin*, the same as in pineapple. It interacts with and activates hydrochloric acid in your stomach. Its action, however, is a little more gentle (not less effective, just not as intense). Now don't immediately assume that because it's not as strong it won't work as well and decide to switch your strawberries to pineapple. Believe me, I know the tricks—I've pulled them all myself. Trust me, nothing you'll do on your own will be more effective than what I tell you to do; you must eat the fruits I tell you to eat, in the order I tell you to eat them, unless, of course, you are allergic to them or really, really hate them. Then you can use the "Substitute Food List" (p. 109). But do not, I repeat, do not replace a required fruit with another just because you like it better or because it worked well for you on other days and *you think it will again.* I can't stress strongly enough the importance of doing everything, and I mean everything, in the designated order.

As you did yesterday, be sure to wait two hours after your last strawberry before you start eating your baked potatoes. In case you've forgotten the waiting rules, I'll go over them one more time. From one fruit to another, wait one hour; from food group to food group, wait two hours. Then again, it would really be a good idea for you to review the "Food Groups" (pp. 113-114) because I'll be talking more about them next week, when I'll be delving more deeply into the technique of Conscious Combining. Believe me, it's important that you understand exactly how this way of eating works in order to be able to adopt it; but don't worry, you will, it's really quite simple.

Let's get back to today's menu and quantities. Most people eat two potatoes, usually the biggest ones they can find. I can't imagine you wanting any more without getting bored, but if you are really still hungry after two, then have more. And yes, you can have butter. However, a word of caution: potatoes are like sponges, they'll soak up as much butter as you give them, so use discretion and try to keep it at about two tablespoons. Likewise, these tasty little "sponges" seem to expand once they're in your stomach, so it's important to eat slowly so you can really tell when you've had enough. If you do eat more than two potatoes, just make sure it's really hunger you are still feeling and not rebellion against authority or "I'll show you."

Yes, I said rebellion. Remember, I've been there too. I've done it all, played every game, pulled every trick. That's why I was fat for 20 years. Once I let go of all those negatives, I became thin. Unfortunately, there was no one to open my eyes to the games I was playing, so it took me longer than it's going to take you. But I'm hopeful that I'll be able to help you see for yourself all those mental and emotional things you're doing to yourself to keep you from being your most perfectly perfect you.

I think most of us already know that being thin does not create a perfect world. It is no panacea. Sorry, being thin won't buy you happiness, but it will do something equally important. It will eliminate the biggest obstacle confronting you today—yourself. As long as your world is colored by "if only's," as long as you stand between you and the person you really want to be, you'll never achieve your full potential or be truly happy. Don't we have enough obstacles in our lives? Aren't there enough things standing between us having and being what we really want?

Do **we** ourselves have to be one of them? But the question is, how do we avoid it? How do we not get caught in that trap? HATING BEING FAT!

You see, for most of us the decision to go on a diet usually comes when we can no longer stand how we look or how we feel. We can only avoid it for so long. Did you ever actually think about what you hate most about being fat or, better yet, what you like the most about being thin? I got in touch with it by making lists, lists that I added to every day. You know, there is much more to getting thin than simply going on a diet. What kept me going, what kept me from saying, "The heck with it," and burying myself under the covers with a cheese and sausage pizza, was to constantly remind myself how much I hated being fat and how great it was going to be to be thin. This little trick, like the many I'm going to share with you, will work miracles.

Actually, I've started your lists for you. On pp. 100 and 101 are lists entitled "What I Hate About Being Fat" and "What's So Great About Being Thin?" Try to add to these lists every day for the next week. Trust me, your entries will serve as inspiration and armor against the fat demon.

You'll see, your entries will stop you from blowing it as nothing else has. In fact, why don't you make your first entry right now, then eat some prunes and have a great day.

D A Y 3

Grapes

I hope you bought a lot of grapes because you're going to need them. You don't have to stop eating at all today, not from the time you get up until the time you to go sleep. Most of us eat about five pounds of grapes on a grape day. Of course, now that I'm thin, I don't have to go on many all-fruit days and neither will you, unless, of course, you want to. For the most part I really only eat fruit to start my day, and since my day starts about 6:00 A.M., by 10 or 11 A.M. I'm famished and will usually have a couple of bagels. That's before lunch, and then I never go back to fruit. Remember, no fruit after another type of food.

Now my lunch could be anything from a plate of broccoli to a hamburger with the works—fries, too! My dinners are even more unpredictable. I eat in restaurants five nights a week and my favorites range from fried calimari and lobster dipped in butter to pasta or prime rib. You, too, will be able to eat this way. The key to it all is the very specific fruits that start your day. Right now, fruit is the catalyst for your weight loss; it is the fruit that allows you to eat foods that are not usually included in a weight-loss program or weight-watching regime.

Your initial weight loss and the effectiveness of my program depends a great deal on the half- and whole-fruit days. However, once you've lost weight, you'll be able to keep it off primarily by beginning every day with fruit. Don't worry if you're a breakfast lover; I'm not going to take your breakfast away from you. You'll just have to get up two hours earlier, eat your fruit, then wait to have the breakfast you love.

Remember, you are not confined to three meals a day when you eat my way. The waiting time of two hours from food group to food group is your only limit and as long as you follow that, you can have as many eating experiences as you desire.

But let's not talk about maintenance yet; let's lose the weight first. And it's already happening, isn't it?

In fact, let's celebrate the weight you have already lost and the weight you're going to lose.

Let's drink a toast to the new soon-to-be-skinny you with a glass of champagne or wine (well, it's the same as grapes, isn't it?), or if you prefer, a glass of ice tea, seltzer or even fruit juice since this is a fruit day. If you choose the wine or champagne, you're not limited to one glass. Alcohol, like food, is not limited in amount. Please keep in mind, however, that you're not eating a lot of heavy food today, so be careful and don't overdo. Getting tipsy—among other things—will pulverize your willpower, so be careful. Alcohol is, of course, optional.

Inasmuch as alcohol is going to be included in your eating scheme (if you wish it to be and you have no problem with it), it's really important for you to study your "Food Groups" (pp. 113-114). Alcohol is like food: you must combine it correctly for it to be non-fattening. Certain types of alcohol combine with certain foods. Wine and champagne come from grapes and you can drink them with fruit. Actually, you can drink champagne with any food because, unlike wine, the bubbles keep it from lingering in your stomach. The grain alcohols—scotch, bourbon, vodka and tequila—go with carbohydrates, as does beer. Again, this is all included in your food group list, so if you are a drinker, please refer to it to see when you'll be able to drink your favorites.

Sorry, no mixers in the drinks. Mixers are what make the drinks fattening. Sparkling or plain water is fine, but no club soda, tonic, cola or other soft drinks, or, heaven forbid, fruit mixes. Unfortunately, this leaves out the tropical drinks, such as margaritas and daiquiris—at least for now!

I hope you've started your Hate-Fat, Love-Thin lists. This, like the other assignments you'll be getting, are very important. (I call them nonphysical exercises.) Trust me when I tell you that they are going to provide you with the impetus and the encouragement when you get discouraged! When you feel as if you can't go on, when all you can focus on are food and eating, pull out these lists and remember your goal.

Believe me, you'll probably have a lot of these moments; it's inevitable. Sticking to a diet and achieving your weight goal are difficult achievements. Nothing you'll ever attempt to do will probably be as tough—but you are going to do it! Just stick with it because there are a lot more tricks up my sleeve. In fact, seeing actress Roseanne on TV talking about her diet reminded me of one of them. She said she and her then-husband, Tom Arnold, were losing weight by eating naked in front of a mirror in the hopes that the sight of themselves in their not-so-glorious "glory" would diminish their appetites. Unlike the Arnolds, I don't ever again want you to look at your body with shame and loathing, no matter how awful it is. So what if your belly touches your thighs like an apron or you can't see your toes. You're thin somewhere! How about your ankles? Have you looked at your hands lately? Come on, don't laugh; I'm serious.

It's time to start accentuating the positive. A thin body won't exist until you can see it. If all you see is the negative, if all you focus on is your fat, then that's all that's going to exist for you. *Well, not anymore!*

At some point today I want you to go stand naked in front of the mirror. I don't care whether you want to or not, just do it! Trust me, you'll live through it. Of course, at first the only thing you are going to see is fat fat fat fat everywhere. . . . Until you look closer. Then, you'll see that not only are there parts of you that aren't bad, there are even some that are kind of nice. If you can't see them right away, look harder. They can be very obscure: the shape of your elbow, the back of your knee. Whatever they are doesn't matter because what starts out as an elbow turns into an arm. The back of the knee flows into the leg. Start looking for your ribs. If you can't see them now, start squiggling around and stretching; you'll catch a glimpse of one sooner or later. Just keep looking and the more time you spend doing it, the sooner it will happen.

Everything—a bridge, a skyscraper, a thin body, a revolution—everything begins with an idea, like your idea that you'll be thin. Reality is nothing more than fantasy realized! *You can make it happen.* Visualize your fantasy body, and you will!

I know, you're worried. You don't think you can make it through a whole day eating nothing but grapes. Of course you can! It's only *one* day. Oh, you think you'll get hungry? How can you get hungry when you can eat as much as you want? Okay, you might get bored, but you certainly won't get hungry. Now you're worried that you might be tempted . . . you won't. Just keep reminding yourself that what's tempting you isn't going anywhere. You'll have the opportunity to eat it another time. Your favorite restaurant won't close and your favorite foods won't disappear. Remember, nothing is leaving the planet— except your FAT!

Tonight, when you drink that toast, make it a birthday toast. HAPPY BIRTHDAY, BORN-AGAIN SKINNY!

D A Y   4

Dried Apricots
Mini Mazel Salad
Pasta

Today is a little more like a normal day, with three very distinct meals. (Although you now know that you aren't limited to eating only three times a day.)

Breakfast, for instance, isn't a one-sitting kind of food. The dried apricots, like the prunes, are something you'll eat start-and-stop, eating them over a period of several hours. Just make sure you eat all eight ounces.

There are various kinds of unsulfured dried apricots to choose from. Some are rather tart, brownish in color, and very dry and chewy. Soaking this kind for about 40 minutes will develop more flavor and make them easier to chew. Again, be sure to drink the water in which they've soaked.

Also, it's important: Don't stop eating your apricots until you've eaten them all—eight ounces exactly.

Dried apricots are going to become an integral part of your diet, not only while you're losing weight, but after you're thin as well. Why are they so important?

For openers, they contain high levels of vitamin A, which is great for your skin, eyes, heart, lungs and liver, as well as mega-amounts of potassium. When it comes to potassium, they have bananas beat by a mile! As I've mentioned earlier, a diet high in potassium will help eliminate bloating. It is also effective in eliminating middle-of-the-night leg cramps. Leg cramps are usually indicative of a potassium deficiency. If you have this problem, you'll find it will probably disappear when you increase your potassium intake.

Before we move on to lunch, let's talk about supplements. If you are already taking some, please continue taking them. Likewise, of course, with any prescription medications. I think vitamin C is always beneficial. I personally take 1,000 to 2,000 mg a day. Taking a high-powered one-a-day multivitamin is also a good idea.

Now let's talk about lunch. First and foremost, be sure to wait two hours after eating your last apricot before you begin lunch. The recipe for the mini Mazel salad is at the end of today's entry. Although it's really meant to be lunch, you may want to save any leftovers in case you get hungry later in the afternoon.

Don't worry about the amount of dressing you use on the salad; you may have as much as you want. If you eat in a restaurant, you can use their oil and vinegar rather than bringing your own.

I told you, eating in a restaurant is no longer an excuse. One by one all of those excuses, along with your fat, are leaving the planet.

Speaking of excuses, we "eaters" are the champion excuse-makers. We can rationalize anything when it comes to eating; any old excuse will do. We reward ourselves with food and we excuse ourselves with food. Whether we're high or low, it really doesn't matter. The end result is the same. The reward becomes the punishment. But the saddest part about it is, all the foods we choose to reward ourselves with are always our favorite foods, the foods we never give ourselves permission to eat when we aren't in an emotional state, when we aren't stressed or hysterical. We never eat them when we are feeling good and can enjoy them. Oh no, the only time we can ever give ourselves permission to eat the things we love is when we're so emotional we can't even enjoy them. These foods, our pleasure-givers, become pain relievers—and create a new pain all their own. Well from now on your reward foods (you know, those foods that you think will make you feel better but never do—beyond, of course, the few seconds they're in your mouth) will be in your Born-Again Skinny weight-loss program and in your slim future. You see all of those open meals coming up? Those are going to be your opportunities to include all the foods you love; foods that will be in your life forever—your soon-to-be-slim forever.

Now, let's get back to today and talk about tonight's dinner. This evening you'll have pasta, pasta, pasta . . . lotsa lotsa pasta. Although I don't want you to go crazy and eat yourself into oblivion, don't stint either; a restaurant portion should be your guide. No, silly— it doesn't have to be plain; you can make marinara sauce, tomato/basil, all'olio or primavera (with vegetables). You can't, however, have cheese or pine nuts because they are proteins. If you make a pesto sauce, you must omit them so the meal remains all carbohydrates. I've also included some recipes, and while you don't have to follow them exactly, at least let them serve as your guide.

If you choose to drink alcohol, remember the rules: champagne goes with anything and most grain alcohols are okay, but check your list. Again, hard liquor goes with carbohydrates; and wine, as you know, goes only with fruit. So if you're a wine drinker, sorry, not tonight; it won't mix. And like everything else, don't try to slip it in or you'll probably gain weight.

Mini Mazel Salad

2 bunches spinach,
    washed thoroughly
3–4 large leeks, cleaned
    and trimmed carefully,
    cut diagonally into
    ¼-inch pieces

20 mushrooms, cleaned
    and sliced
Mazel dressing

Combine vegetables. Toss with Mazel dressing (p. 131).

YIELD: 2 servings

Pasta with Olive Oil and Garlic

1 pound spaghetti,
  fettuccine or linguini
½ cup olive oil, plus oil
  for cooking water

2–3 large cloves garlic,
  peeled and minced
Freshly ground black
  pepper

Cook pasta in several quarts of boiling water with a few drops of oil. Cook al dente and drain thoroughly.

Heat oil and toss in cooked pasta. Cook 1–2 minutes over medium low heat. Toss in garlic* and cook 30 seconds over low heat. Do not brown garlic. Add a few grindings of fresh pepper.

YIELD: 2 servings

Pasta with Sautéed Vegetables

8 large mushrooms,
  cleaned and sliced
½ cup, plus 2 tablespoons
  olive oil
10 broccoli florets,
  blanched 2 minutes and
  refreshed**

10 asparagus spears, cut
  diagonally, blanched
  2 minutes and refreshed
1 pound spaghetti, cooked***
  and drained
2 large cloves garlic, minced
Freshly ground black pepper

* Some cooks recommend sautéing the garlic in oil first. If you do sauté it, use caution and don't brown it, or it will be bitter. Cook only until slightly golden; then add to pasta.
** To "refresh" means to rinse under cold water.
*** Some people cook the pasta in the water the vegetables have been cooked in.

Sauté mushrooms in 1 tablespoon hot oil 1–2 minutes. Set aside. Sauté broccoli 1 minute in 1½ teaspoons hot oil. Sauté asparagus 1 minute in 1½ teaspoons hot oil.

Heat ½ cup oil. Sauté pasta 1–2 minutes. Add vegetables and garlic and cook 1 minute. Add pepper and serve.

YIELD: 2 servings

Pasta with Peas

1 cup onions, finely
  chopped
¼ cup butter
¼ cup olive oil
2 cloves garlic, finely
  chopped
6 ounces large pasta
  shells, cooked and
  drained

10 ounces small pasta
  shells, cooked and
  drained
2½ cups cooked peas
1 cup parsley, finely
  chopped
Freshly ground black
  pepper

Sauté onions in combination of butter and oil 6–8 minutes. Add garlic and cook very slowly for another moment or two. Remove from heat and add shells, peas, parsley and pepper. Mix well to serve.

YIELD: 2 servings

D A Y 5

Pineapple
Papaya
Pineapple

Whenever I think of today, I can't help but hear the song "Rawhide"—I change the words a little but the gist is still the same: Burn 'em up, move 'em out, enzymes, trusty enzymes.

There are probably no two fruits with more potent enzymes than pineapples and papayas. It was shortly after I began applying the age-old principles of food combining to my diet that I discovered their potential. More than just delicious, they actually spelled the difference between *fat and thin.*

Pineapple contains the powerful fat-burning enzyme bromelin. I mentioned it earlier, on your strawberry day. Remember, it interacts with and activates hydrochloric acid in your stomach. It is your "natural" fat digester. Your fat digester, by the way, is chiefly responsible for breaking down all the dairy products you eat—milk, cheese, yogurt, ice cream, butter—the meat and fowl you eat and (the real killers) the snacks you munch on—cookies, chips, crackers and pretzels made with *hydrogenated* or *partially hydrogenated* oil, etc.

Start reading the labels and start replacing your snack items with more healthful varieties made with "good" oils, such as safflower or canola. Look for these products in the natural foods sections of most large grocery stores or at your local health food store. Just remember, no matter where you are, always read the labels. Make sure the foods you buy don't contain hydrogenated or partially hydrogenated oil. Hydrogenated and partially hydrogenated oils are solid at room temperature. The hydrogenated and partially hydrogenated fats are what have given the food group "fats" their much undeserved bad reputation.

Papaya, your other fruit for today, is equally powerful. I haven't told you yet about the *bam bam bam* of the papaya. Just like a little hammer, it pounds away at that surplus flesh and excess fat and softens it so that your body can eliminate it. See what I mean by burn 'em up, move 'em out, enzymes? For the next couple of days we are really going to be attacking those fat deposits.

The enzyme in papaya is *papain;* the natural enzyme in your body that papaya gives a boost to is pepsin. Papain in a chemical or man-made form is used as an ingredient in meat tenderizer.

It's important to eat your fruit today in the exact order I specified—that is, if you want to "burn 'em up and move 'em out, enzymes."

Eat pineapple until you just can't eat anymore (at

least a whole one), then wait one hour and eat papaya until you think you'll turn into one (at least two or three). After you've stopped for at least an hour, eat more pineapple.

If your mouth hurts from the pineapple, it's probably because it's not ripe. If you are lucky enough to have a market that sells halved or skinned pineapples, that is your safest choice. You can see what you're getting and leave nothing to chance. If you are going to buy whole pineapples, let me give you a few easy tips: A ripe uncut pineapple should be golden yellow with a flowery, fragrant and sweet aroma. It should smell like a pineapple. Your nose, by the way, is your best guide to ripe fruit. Color and texture can be misleading, but not your nose. If fruit doesn't smell, it won't taste. This, by the way, also applies to vegetables, especially tomatoes. However, with watermelon and grapes, it's not that easy, but you can pick a ripe watermelon by its sound. Turn it over so its belly—the underside—is on top. Take your fist and knock it across that area. If it's a high "ping," it's not ripe. If it's a deep "thump," it's overripe. A perfect watermelon will be a resounding "boom."

Grapes don't really smell, so you'll have to eyeball them. In the old days before Conscious Combining, I'd snatch a sample, but not anymore. You know, it's not the binges or fancy meals that make you fat, it's the things that, as the late Totie Fields used to say, ". . . fly into your mouth." So when it comes to selecting fruit, or any "tasting" for that matter, if you catch yourself in mid-bite, don't swallow it. Discreetly spit it out. Remember, for every bite that goes in your mouth, something else can't. Every bite, no matter how small, counts. So when that little voice says, "Should I or shouldn't I . . .?" and you're about to take that first mouthful, ask yourself if that bite is worth giving up another bite that is yet to come. In other words, if you think about food when it doesn't count, you won't have to think about it when it does.

DAY 6

Papaya
Steak or Lamb Chops, and Shrimp, Any Style

L et's keep that hammer pounding a while longer: at least three more papayas are in store for you today. More, of course, if you'd like. Just eat your little heart out. Again, don't make yourself sick by overeating, but remember that with these enzymatic fruits, the more you eat the more you'll lose.

When people complain that they don't feel well or that they feel weak or tired, it's often because they haven't eaten enough. Don't let that happen to you, especially today because I want you feeling great tonight, particularly if you're going out to your favorite steak house. If you don't eat red meat, you can have the animal protein of your choice—fish, fowl or pork. If you are a vegetarian, eat whatever you would normally eat for protein.

If you're cooking at home, I hope you've selected your favorite cut of steak. Always be sure to give yourself the *best* of your *favorites* in order to really seal in your success. One of the reasons we lose control is because we become frustrated when we haven't eaten what we really wanted to eat. We give ourselves permission to break our diet and eat something we think we shouldn't be eating—such as a pizza, a banana split or nachos with extra cheese—and yet we don't fully indulge ourselves by going to our favorite pizza spot or ice cream parlor or hamburger joint. Instead of feeding ourselves our fantasy—our ultimate favorite burger or ice cream or Mexican food—we'll have it just anywhere and prepared any way. Usually the faster we get the food, the better. We want to eat it before our skinny person regains control and we decide to skip it.

So meanwhile, we have this inferior "cheat treat," and all it does is cause more dissatisfaction and frustration because it doesn't compare. It's not nearly as good as your favorite, that to which you're comparing it. Then what happens is you wind up still wanting more—more of just *anything* to fill that void of dissatisfaction.

When it comes to pizza, spareribs or bacon-cheeseburgers, it's rare you'll see me eating them anywhere other than my favorite places.

Choosing the best fruit is equally important. Making sure that it's ripe and eating it before it gets overripe are critical to your success, so don't shop for fruit too far in advance. You'll only hurt yourself—it won't taste good and you won't be satisfied.

As always, there is no portion control tonight. (And yes, you can use cocktail sauce with your shrimp or ketchup on your steak.) Go easy on the condiments, though; they are apt to be salty. Avoid steak sauce for this same reason. If, however, you can find one that is salt- and MSG-free, eat your heart out. No butter or oil, please: they're not necessary with meat, and will make it less healthful.

Yes, meat can be healthful when properly cooked and eaten in moderation, certainly not seven days a week. Even the fat can be a necessary nutritional component. Contrary to what you may think, we need fat in our diets. Among other things, fat transports hormones as well as vitamins A, D, E and K, and replenishes the cells in the sheaths surrounding nerves.

If your doctor has advised you not to eat meat, follow your doctor's instructions. Again, if you're a vegetarian, eat whatever you would normally eat for protein, but beware of cheese. It's very hard to digest, and if you are eating a lot of it, it probably bears most of the responsibility for those unwanted pounds.

If you're drinking alcohol, it's champagne only tonight.

DAY 7

Pineapple Mazel Salad

Day number seven and you're in heaven, and why not? Not only did you stick to your diet all week, not only did you not cheat once, but you lost weight . . . and it wasn't even hard.

Well, how difficult was it to eat corn on the cob and baked potatoes, pasta and steak? Next week is even better. Your favorite meal, a sandwich, chicken and turkey (as much as you like, skin and all, dark meat or white) plus a Chinese banquet. Not too shabby!

If you can eat this way and lose weight, imagine how easy it will be to maintain your weight! That's right: this technique is going to allow you to eat whatever you want and never gain weight. So what if you have to eat a lot of sweet, delicious, fat-burning pineapple in the process? It certainly beats a liquid chemical in a can or two ounces of this and a half cup of that—your basic calorie-counting, portion control, starve-yourself diet.

I really want you to eat a lot of pineapple today, so don't hold back. Let's put those enzymes to work.

I hope you're looking forward to your salad tonight because awaiting you is a salad the likes of which you've never tasted before. It's the combination of ingredients that creates its zip, both in your mouth and in your body, so use as many, if not all, of the ingredients as possible.

If you've been a little edgy or feeling as if you wanted to blow it, it's only natural! Sticking to a diet—any diet—is tough, and I'm sure there will be many days when you don't think you can make it. Think of all the temptations: the smells, all those food commercials, packing the kids' lunches, fixing the family dinner. How many times did you catch yourself with a food in your mouth you weren't supposed to be eating? I hope you didn't swallow it.

You know it is funny: we really don't think we eat differently than other people. Oh sure, we have our moments of madness when our head says no and our heart says go, and off we go, eating everything that isn't nailed down. But forget about the binges; the truth of the matter is we *do* eat more, and differently, than the so-called "normal" or, shall we say, skinny person. We just don't realize it because we're not aware of it. What I'm talking about is unconscious eating. Recall what I said yesterday, how it's not the fancy meals or the big blowouts that get us. It's all the eating we do when we aren't really eating, the bites of this, the nibbles of that, the hard candy we pick up at the dry cleaners, the leftovers as we clear the table.

This need that we have to eat, however, is as inherent in our personalities and is as much a part of us as any other character trait that we have. That's why I'll never ask you to change or eliminate your urge to eat, but rather to be aware of it and learn how to turn it into a positive force. You can make it work for you instead of against you. If you make every bite count and think about food when it doesn't count, you won't have to think about it when it does.

For every bite that goes in your mouth, something else can't. The bites we have to be the most aware of are the ones we don't even know we've had, like the "meal" before the meal.

The next time you cook for someone other than yourself, be aware of how often you almost stick something in your mouth—your finger, a spoon . . . Although your seven days on *The New Beverly Hills Diet* have made you aware of everything that goes in your mouth, I'm sure on more than one occasion you'll find yourself unconsciously putting something in your mouth that does not belong there. Stay on guard; old habits die hard.

Mazel Salad

2 bunches spinach,
    washed thoroughly
2 bunches watercress
2 small heads Belgian
    endive
1–2 bunches mustard
    greens
3 carrots, grated
2 raw beets, grated

1 Daikon radish, grated
25 mushrooms, cleaned
    and sliced
1 bunch chopped parsley
3 leeks, cleaned and
    trimmed carefully, cut
    diagonally into $1/4$-inch
    pieces
Mazel dressing

Be sure all vegetables are clean and thoroughly dry. Tear spinach, watercress, endive and mustard greens into large, bite-sized pieces. Add remaining ingredients. Toss with Mazel dressing (p. 131).

YIELD: 2 servings

DAY 8

Grapes
(Raisins or Popcorn Optional)

Another Monday and a thinner you. Now, when people start noticing those lost pounds, be sure to smile and say thank you. Tomorrow you'll probably also be saying thank you to your scale. You'll usually experience a loss after a grape day, despite the fact that you should have eaten at least five pounds of grapes.

I love red grapes, especially frozen. Just pop them in your freezer for a couple of hours and you'll have a real taste treat—and a little diversion.

If it's cherry season and you prefer cherries instead of grapes—indulge. Just be sure that you're eating cherries in place of, *not in addition to,* grapes. But please, don't swallow those hard little pits, and be sure the cherries are nice and ripe or you'll get a stomach ache. Their deep color will be the key. Whether your choice is cherries or grapes, you can have four ounces of raisins *or* a large bowl of popcorn tonight. If you choose popcorn, don't forget to wait the two hours; one hour for raisins. You can cook the popcorn in oil, but please, no butter or salt. In the future, you'll be able to jazz it up with butter, but not tonight. Tonight we're using that popcorn as a broom. We want it to sweep, and butter will only slow it down. A word of warning: don't use packaged microwave popcorn; it's loaded with artificial ingredients.

Have you and your bathroom scale become friends yet? That little mechanical device has more effect on us than an atom bomb. It can literally make or break our day. Well, you aren't alone if you hate it. It can take the strongest of egos and shatter it to smithereens. I have seen the most gorgeous, the most powerful, the most secure and the most self-assured crumble beneath its force. The scale, along with food, represents our enemy (or should I say, former enemy?).

The scale forces us to see and feel ourselves as we really are, and it forces us to do something about it. If you had really seen yourself as you were, would you have let yourself look the way you did? If you had really felt yourself, don't you think you would have done something about it long before now? How easy was it to carry that heavy watermelon from the check-out stand to your car? How easy was it to carry around all those extra pounds? If you had really been conscious of them you would have done something about it. The scale forces us into consciousness.

No matter how evolved we become, no matter how thin we get, we retain an investment in disconnecting from our bodies, a vestige of what I call our mind/body split. We see what we want to see, and we feel what we want to feel. When we look in the mirror, we have a preconceived idea of what we look like and that is what we see . . .

The first trip I went on after I became a Skinny was to New York City for nine days. Remember, I used to weigh 180 pounds. There I was, a new Skinny without my scale, away from my farmer's market, being wined and dined. Would my technique of Conscious Combining really work? Would it pass the test out there in the "real world"? I was scared! Then I arrived at the hotel and discovered a scale in my room. What a relief! Each night I celebrated eating while still following my rules, and each morning I weighed myself. Conscious Combining was working. I was thrilled! My weight never wavered.

One night, I gave myself permission to really splurge, or do what I call an "open without discretion," and I dined in grand style. It was an open Italian and I mixed it all: grease, cheese and salt. I had tried to eat like a skinny person—slowly, consciously, one bite at a time—but I lost control, I went overboard. I was sure I had gained.

The next morning I could feel it as I rolled out of bed. I looked in the mirror: my hipbones had vanished. I had really done it this time. I was terrified. The whale that I once was loomed before me. I inched onto the scale with dread and horror. With one eye shut, barely breathing, I looked down. Three numbers stared up at me. *Three perfect numbers.* I had not gained an ounce! I had succeeded. I had eaten like a thin person, with one hand, one bite at a time, and despite my "open without discretion," despite my being out of control, I hadn't gained a pound. I didn't have to be afraid anymore; I could schedule open days more often. Overcome with joy and relief, I looked in the mirror again. My hipbones reappeared. My mind had been playing tricks on me; the scale brought reality back into focus.

What a sense of security the scale affords! From that moment on I haven't traveled without one. I have a very small, lightweight bathroom scale that slips easily into the bottom of my suitcase.

Your scale is your best friend; it's your nonjudgmental lover. It is the one truly objective observer in your life. It has no ulterior motives. Most important, it no longer tells you if you've been good or bad, but rather, if what you are doing and what you are eating are working or not working. And if it's not working, if you've gained a little, big deal; it's not the end of the world. It doesn't mean that you should get hysterical and beat yourself over the head because you are a fat failure. It doesn't mean that you'll never again be able to eat whatever it was you ate that made you gain. It means that you'll make it work. That is what *The New Beverly Hills Diet* program is all about. Making food, all food, regardless of its inevitable and transitory effect, work. So if the scale is up, you'll simply apply the rules of Conscious Compensation, use the corrective counterparts and eat your way back down. You'll get thin by feeding your body, and you'll stay thin by feeding your body.

On this program you'll be experimenting with food to see what does and doesn't work for you. The scale is there to tell you exactly how much you can get away with. This is a learning experience that can only happen if you commit yourself to a daily love affair with your scale.

The worst thing you can do is not weigh yourself after you blow it . . . spend the day feeling fat and guilty when perhaps you didn't even gain any weight. Keep in mind that it's not the big meals that get you, it's not the indiscretions you've planned for or those "moments of madness," it's all the things you think really don't matter (like the lick off a spoon you used to stir something). Let the scale prove it to you.

Confront and acknowledge your weight every day. Then, let it go. Weigh yourself every day, write it down, and tell it to the same person. Erase that fat consciousness once and for all. If you do not confront and acknowledge your weight, it hangs around. Jackie, one of my clients, used to tell me her weight in code. She'd write down 10 pounds less than it was, and when she called her weight in each day, she'd only give the last digit. She thought her husband, Henry, had no idea what she weighed. Then she got stuck on a plateau. Nothing was working. Her weight remained at the same maddening number. Of course, I felt that if she would admit her weight, the plateau would dissolve. Yet nothing could persuade her, not even the thought of three watermelon days in succession.

Finally, in desperation, I asked her to put her husband on the phone. She consented. "How much do you think Jackie weighs, Henry?" Despite her code, despite her dressing in the closet to hide her fat, despite every ploy known only to the fat, Henry guessed Jackie's weight within a pound.

Once Jackie realized that her weight wasn't a secret, and once she herself said it aloud, she lost three pounds. The plateau had been mental, not physical.

Love your scale and embrace it; it is one of the keys to your success and your foundation to your sense of being. It will make this diet work for you, and it will make food and eating work for you. It will get you skinny and keep you skinny if only you allow it.

What have you got to lose?

DAY 9

Prunes
Strawberries
Chicken or Turkey

There is a little more variety today than yesterday . . . three different foods. Prunes are first. As always, eat eight ounces. Wait one hour before starting your strawberries and eat a lot of them. Remember, the more you eat the more you lose. You might try putting some in a blender with a little ice and making a drink out of them. Actually, you can do this with any of the fruits for a little change of pace. Cooking them is also great. I'll tell you how to do that tomorrow. You just might want to bake your pineapple—mmmmm, good.

Have you decided on tonight's dinner yet? Is it going to be chicken or turkey or both? To tell you the truth, choosing one or the other over having some of both would be better, but if you really want variety, it's fine to have some of each. You can even have dark meat and, yes, you can eat the skin.

The reason it's better to choose one or the other is that it diminishes the tendency to overeat. It's important for those of us who never seem to know when enough is enough, for those of us who are ruled by our taste buds, not our stomachs. Choosing the Mono-Meal (eating one thing at a time) is our savior. When you're eating only one thing, you really can't do much serious damage, weight-wise, because you will ultimately eat considerably less than you would if you had eaten a mixture of foods. For some of us, our stomachs almost never say "enough," and as long as the food continues to taste good, we can still fit more in no matter how stuffed we are! You see, when you eat a variety of things at one time, you trigger off a variety of taste buds, and even when your stomach has had quite enough, your taste buds greedily ask for more. However, when you stick to one thing, sooner or later those taste buds get bored and hopefully when it stops tasting good, you'll stop eating. That usually happens before you've seriously overeaten.

I know I've already spoken at length about exercise, and you know it's not compulsory. However, if you have a regular routine, I hope you've continued doing it, provided you don't work out with weights.

I don't want you to use weights now because I don't want you to build up any muscle mass, nor do I want you to change fat into muscle. The fruits you are eating are helping soften all your surplus flesh so we can get it off. We don't want to lock it in. Don't worry, you'll firm up when your weight is where it should be.

Now I know I told you I wasn't going to make you exercise and I'm still not, but if you're one of those people that do nothing physical at all and exercise has not been a part of your life up to now, I'm going to ask you to take a first step. I want you to do a little something physical for five minutes a day. Come on, five minutes is no big deal. You have a choice: turn on the radio and dance nonstop for five minutes, or take a walk around the block. If you don't want to leave home, then walk in place for five minutes.

What good will five minutes do? When your body is used to doing nothing, just doing something (even a little something) will add some fire to the furnace we're trying to charge up. That furnace, by the way, is called your metabolism.

So, if your excuse has always been your "slow metabolism," it won't be slow for long. You're changing all of that now that you're feeding your body the highest octane gasoline, and you're going to see a dramatic change in pace.

D A Y 1 0

Dried Apricots
Papaya
Pineapple

Today is an interesting day: all fruit, but taste and texture-wise, each fruit is delightfully and deliciously individual and each has its own jobs. As you recall, the apricots are primarily for potassium. Adding potassium in its natural food form (pure food is always more potent than pills) will keep you from retaining water. This will be important to remember when you start planning your own menus. You'll find that if you have dried apricots for breakfast on a day in which you know you are going to have a very salty meal (Chinese or Japanese food, for instance), the extra potassium will help fend off any bloating.

The papaya is softening that extra "meat" on your bones, so eat at least two or three of them. Last but not least is pineapple. Please eat at least a whole one. Pineapple will burn up what the papaya has softened. We're getting that fat ready for the watermelon to wash it out tomorrow.

If you want to try something different with your pineapple tonight, why not make a drink out of it? Or if you're just dying for something hot, cut the pineapple in half lengthwise, sprinkle cinnamon on the yellow part and place it skin-side down in a baking dish with a little water. Put it in a pre-heated 400° oven and immediately turn the oven down to 225°. Bake for about two or three hours, or until the fragrant aroma of pineapple wafts through your house. You can also do this with papayas, bananas and strawberries for a little variety. Just remember, preheat the oven to a high heat and then lower the setting when you put in your fruit.

It's been 10 days since you've started the program, so I'm sure you have had to face at least once social situation. They're always hard at first, particularly the way you're now eating. It's hard to be inconspicuous when all you're eating is watermelon or grapes. Besides, most restaurants don't have these items on their menus. (Well, they didn't have them on the menus in Beverly Hills 16 years ago either; at least not until people started asking for them.) I know it's hard trying to have a social life while sticking to a diet. First of all, who wants to admit that they're on a diet? Then they'd be admitting they're fat (as if the rest of the world hadn't already noticed; trust me, long, big jackets only hide so much).

Do not, I repeat, DO NOT under any circumstances, make any social sacrifices even while you are on this early, somewhat strict and very specific phase of the program. It's important to experience eating out in the real world from the very beginning. Only then can you really begin to make conscious food choices in your natural environment. Right now you'll just have to go with the flow and eat what you are supposed to eat no matter what, even if it means going to your favorite restaurant and watching your friends eat your favorite foods while you are eating grapes. You'll learn that all the food that passes before you will still be there tomorrow. You only know it tastes good because you have eaten it before and you'll eat it again. Realizing this and remembering this will be important to your slim future because, let's face it, even when you're thin there will be times that you'll have to remind yourself that enough is enough.

If you're feeling a little unsure of yourself, practice your restaurant dialogue in front of a mirror. Act out telling the waiter or waitress that you are on a special diet. Let him or her know that you can only eat watermelon or whatever it is you are eating that day. Mention that you've brought your own with you and ask for a plate.

I know it seems hard at first, but trust me when I tell you that the world understands, and most people only wish they had your courage and strength—the courage and strength that continue to increase day by day.

D A Y 1 1

Watermelon

You may think watermelon is nothing but water, right? Well, you're wrong. It is high in trace minerals, chlorine, bromine, sulfur, potassium and even protein. Most important, it is literally going to help flush out all the fat we've been burning up over the past 10 days. I love to eat the seeds and, contrary to what your mother told you, a watermelon will not grow in your stomach if you do so. Just be sure to chew them before you swallow them.

I think seeds are the most important part of any fruit. They're the source of the nutrients and the focus of the enzymes. They're the living, breathing part of the fruit. If you plant them, they'll grow (but not in your stomach). They are energy, pure and simple. When something has seeds, such as watermelon, grapes or papayas, try to eat a few of them. Papaya seeds are interesting. They taste somewhat like capers and are very peppery.

Now, back to the watermelon. Eat a lot of it. Cut it up so you can carry it with you, or eat it Buddy Hackett-style. . . . A former client of mine, Buddy taught me a thing or two about watermelon. He had a very interesting technique. He'd take his whole watermelon and cut a little cap-like slice off the top, then he'd hold the whole thing in the crook of his arm and scoop it out with a spoon while sitting in an easy chair. (I could tell you my Jack Nicholson watermelon story, but I don't want to embarrass you.)

DAY 12

Dried Apricots
Avocado Sandwich
Three Veggies with Rice

Your breakfast of dried apricots will replace any potassium you may have lost yesterday on your watermelon day. Watermelon is a wonderful natural diuretic, promoting, as you may have noticed, frequent urination.

What is it about eating a sandwich that we love so much? Can it be the look of it, the way it feels in our hands, the sensation of biting into it, the taste and textures? Well, you tell me tomorrow after you have experienced one and have continued to lose weight to boot. It's hard to believe that you can even eat a sandwich on a diet, and look at what kind of a sandwich it is.

I know you're thinking that avocados are so fattening. True, they can be, but not when they are combined correctly with other foods.

You can have your sandwich on any type of bread or roll, with tomato, onion, sprouts and lettuce. Of course, you can use sour cream or even mayonnaise, preferably homemade or the health food store variety without preservatives. The recipe for homemade is at the end of today's entry. You can make the sandwich as large as you want. I love mine with all the fixin's sliding out the sides. To me, that's half the fun of eating it. You'll notice that avocados are either/or's— they combine with proteins or carbohydrates, but never both.

Dinner tonight is what we call in *The New Beverly Hills Diet* talk an "open carb meal." That's a meal that is all carbohydrates. Carbohydrates are the nutrients that supply your body with energy.

Tonight is actually a good night for a Chinese feast . . . stir-fry veggies and vegetable fried rice. You have your choice of any three vegetables, cooked any way you'd like. You can eat them with any kind of rice; the choice is up to you. Don't use salt or anything containing salt, such as soy sauce or MSG. If you go to a Chinese restaurant, be sure to tell them what NOT to use in preparing your meal. If you use butter or oil, use discretion. Two tablespoons should be quite enough. Some people might say "in moderation," but not I; that's another word I don't like because I'm not good at practicing it, especially when it comes to eating. I may be thin but I'm an "eater," and you know how we "eaters" are: if something is good, more is better, too much is not enough, and I want it all.

Now, what I'd like you to do is turn to p. 113 so we can go through the "Food Groups" together. As you see, there are five food group headings: fruit, proteins, fats, carbohydrates, and either/ors. Under each category is listed a variety of foods that fall into the individual categories. All foods contain some protein, some carbohydrates and some fats. Fruit, although listed separately, is actually a carbohydrate. However, it is a carbohydrate in a category all its own because it must be eaten alone. It should not be eaten with anything else, not even other carbohydrates.

You'll remember that a food is classified according to its major components. Carbohydrates are at least 51 percent glucose; proteins, 51 percent amino acids; and fats, 51 percent lipids. All are equally important and none is more fattening than the other. It is the proper balance of all food groups in our diets that will keep us slim and healthy. Balanced, as I said earlier, not daily, but weekly.

Carbohydrates comprise the majority of the foods we eat, so we'll start with them.

Every vegetable from an artichoke to a zucchini is a carbohydrate, as are potatoes, grains, bread, pasta and cereal. I'm not sure when or why people stopped thinking of the lighter vegetables (lettuce, chard, kale, parsley) as carbohydrates, but they are, indeed. I call them *mini-carbs*. There are different types of carbohydrates. The difference is based on their molecular structure. The maxi-carb (or starch) is the most complex and requires the longest time to digest. But don't let that frighten you. It doesn't mean maxi-carbs are more fattening. Mini-carb or maxi-carb, it's the same four calories per gram. Forget what you've been hearing about carbohydrate sensitivity. Eaten correctly, they will not make you fat. But then you should already know that, you've eaten enough carbs in the past 10 days to beat the band (pasta, potatoes, rice, corn on the cob), not to mention all that fruit (also carbohydrates). What more proof do you need? Have you gained or lost weight? **Food is fattening when it is not processed or digested efficiently,** when it becomes trapped in our stomachs longer than it should either because of enzyme interference or when faster-digesting foods are eaten with slower-digesting foods.

Fruit is the fastest digesting food of all. Unlike all other foods, fruit does not require much help from our stomachs to digest; it should be in and out in the form of nutrients almost instantly. For instance, before you can finish eating your pineapple, some of its nutrients are already nourishing your cells. Problems arise when we eat fruit *with* other foods or *after* other foods. That fruit will get trapped and just sit in our stomachs as it rots. (Well, what would happen if you took a piece of fruit and put it in a room that was over 100°? It would ferment, of course. That's what happens to fruit in our stomachs when it is eaten with or after other foods.) Stop for a minute and think back to how often you felt bloated after eating fruit in the middle of the day or as a dessert.

To be nonfattening and efficiently utilized by your body, fruit must be eaten alone and never after any other type of food. **Remember, once you have eaten any other type of food in the course of the day, you never, ever eat fruit again that day (no matter how many hours have elapsed).**

Now let's talk about the other carbs, starting with the maxis (starches). Please, don't look at the maxi-carb list with fear and horror. Remember, maxi or mini, they all have the same four calories per gram. Maxi-carbs are the carbohydrates that provide your body with maximum, long-acting sustained energy and they, like all other carbohydrates, are only potentially fattening when they are inefficiently digested, when they are trapped in your stomach with proteins (a slower-digesting food) or when they are eaten after a protein, when the key carbohydrate-digesting enzyme ptyalin is annihilated by the combination of the protein-digesting enzymes. Proteins spend a long time in your stomach—about six hours for fish, for example, but much longer for chicken and beef. Bear in mind that as long as your stomach is working on protein, any carbohydrate you eat thereafter will not only sit like a lump in your stomach waiting for that protein to get out, it will be a lump that has not been predigested because the ptyalin that should have been in your saliva was not there.

Fats go with proteins or carbohydrates, but never with fruit (but then, nothing ever goes with fruit). *Please*, you must stop thinking of fats as a four-letter word. They are essential to good health.

The last food group is the either/or's—the beans and avocado. I call them either/or's because they take on the characteristics of the food group with which they are eaten. They are protein when consumed with protein and carbohydrates when consumed with carbohydrates. They can be mixed with proteins or carbohydrates, but never with both at the same time, lest you want bricks and mortar.

Mazel Mayonnaise

1 whole egg
1 egg yolk
1/4 – 1/2 teaspoon dry
   mustard (use more or
   less, to taste)

3 teaspoons rice vinegar
2 cups sesame oil

In a small bowl, whisk together egg, egg yolk, mustard and vinegar. Whisk in 1/2 cup of the oil, 1 tablespoon at a time, whisking thoroughly as you go to ensure emulsification. Add remaining oil in a thin stream until mixture is thick and smooth. May be thinned with water. (You can also prepare this mayonnaise in a food processor or blender.)

YIELD: approx. 2 cups

D A Y   1 3

Grapes
Two Bananas

Iknow that there are many of you who read my first book and went on my diet. As you can see, although some of the foods you have been eating are the same foods you ate before and there still are, like today, some all-fruit days, *The New Beverly Hills Diet* is far more liberal and there is much more food in many more miscombinations. That's the real treat.

The original rules of Conscious Combining—protein with protein, carbohydrates with carbohydrates, fruit alone—were not written in stone. That's how we would eat if this were an ideal world, but we live in the real world. And the reality is a hamburger with everything on it . . . without the patty is okay once in a while, but it's only a substitute for the real thing. Sooner or later you want that patty. To a meat loaf lover, what's meat loaf without the mashed potatoes? So asking you to spend the rest of your life never mixing foods is no different or better than asking you to count calories or weigh and measure your portions. It's not realistic and you'd never stick to it. Through my experiments over the last 15 years, I've come to discover that total abstinence from mixing foods is not 100 percent necessary, and everyone should ultimately be able to get away with at least one miscombination a day. Some people can even get away with two a day. A miscombination is a meal combining proteins and carbohydrates.

How many miscombinations will you personally be able to get away with? Let me ask you this: How many will you want to get away with? Your weight isn't the only consideration. Remember, when you mix foods you are not reaping their full nutritional value nor are you experiencing their full energy-giving potential. Food is your energy. You are a product of what you eat, pure and simple. You have to think not only about how you react sensually to food, but also how you react physically to food. How you feel, how you look, how people relate to you, and how your life does or doesn't work for you all depend on your energy. Your energy is a magnet, drawing back to you whatever you put out, and that energy comes from one source: the food you eat. Food is your life and your life depends on it.

When I choose not to miscombine, it's usually not because it's going to make me fat, but rather because I'm not going to feel so great after I do.

All the fruit you've been eating and the isolation of the food groups have heightened your awareness and sensitivity. As we begin reintegrating some mixed meals back into your diet, I'm sure you'll see what I mean or, rather, you'll feel what I mean. It just doesn't feel as good.

When it comes to weight loss, the number of miscombinations you'll be able to get away with each week has to do with you and your ability to know when enough is enough. This is an area in which most "eaters" have a problem. So, it is imperative that you stay conscious of miscombinations. Actually, it's not as hard as it sounds. When you know that it is permissible to have a chocolate soufflé any day of the week, you don't have to eat three times as much as you need. When you are on an eating program that allows you to go out and enjoy that Sunday champagne brunch, dessert table and all, every Sunday, then every time you go to a buffet it doesn't mean you have to go crazy and eat yourself into oblivion.

There are several keys to successfully mixing food. The waiting time is one of them. As long as you wait the appropriate time between foods and food groups, you are not confined to three meals a day. Starting your day with fruit is crucial; in fact, its effect is so dramatic that if you do nothing else but begin every day with the enzymatic fruits you've been eating these past days, you'll be pounds ahead of the weight game. This alone will help you from ever returning to your former fat self. Obviously, that's not all there is to it. Eating the fruit in the morning will keep your body reasonably controlled; Conscious Combining will keep it totally controlled.

If you only have one miscombination meal a day, no matter how bad it is (combination-wise), you'll also never get fat again if you have eaten your morning fruit and then limit or exclude the carbohydrates you eat for the rest of that day. Remember the 80 percent Protein Rule.

Once you have had your protein/carbohydrate combination for the day (steak and baked potato, or pizza, for example), you must look at every carbohydrate as the enemy because, I repeat, once protein is in your stomach, the carbohydrate-digesting enzyme, ptyalin, is annihilated and that carbohydrate is going to sit in your stomach waiting for the protein to get out. Knowing that, you must always ask yourself if you still really want that carb. Well you're only human, and I'm sure situations will arise when you will. So it is then that you must really use discretion when eating another miscombination meal containing more carbohydrates. Then, those carbohydrates should not exceed more than 20 percent of the total meal. In other words, any meal following a miscombined meal should be at least 80 percent (if not all) protein, or you'll soon be back in Fat City.

D A Y 1 4

Pineapple
Strawberries
Open with Discretion

Here it is, your third Sunday on a diet! I know you actually started your diet two Mondays ago and tomorrow will really only be two weeks, but you really have to count the day before you started. That was the *last time* you selected a meal on your own. Well, did you behave any differently that night than any other night before a new diet? Isn't it always the same the night before you start a new diet? Don't you have to eat everything you think you're never going to eat again? You probably thought this diet was just more of the same, just another diet you'd stick to until you became bored. I'm sure by now you must realize that this is an all-new ball game. This isn't just another diet.

And now it's time to put into action the Skinny consciousness you're developing. True, tonight you're on your own, just as you were only two short weeks ago. However, unlike that night, you won't be eating with guilt and remorse, ever fearful of the fat consequences

of your food folly. Tonight, you'll be eating with permission and with pleasure. I'm not going to tell you
what to eat or how much. You can eat whatever you
would like, your heart's desire whatever that may be.
The amount? Let your conscience (your Skinny conscience, that is) be your guide. The "fat you" always
overdid it in the past; that's why you are on a diet now.
Well, you don't have to overdo anymore because any of
the foods you choose to eat, those you've always
overeaten in the past, are not being taken away from
you. You don't have to eat them all, try to cram every
last one in or eat yourself under the table. It's not the
last time you'll get to eat them. It's only the first time,
the first time of many. These foods are on your individual eating program forever and they're not going to
disappear. So use discretion when you eat and eat like
a human being, with one hand, one bite at a time,
aware of the tastes and the textures, and how the food
feels going down your throat. Remind yourself that it's
not how much you eat in how short a time, but how
long you can make the pleasure last!

The pineapple and strawberries that make up
today's menu will prepare your body with fat-burning
enzymes, high-level nutrition and high-octane fuel.
They'll help your body digest whatever you may give
it tonight, no matter how badly you miscombine (I
don't care if it's eggplant parmigiana and Italian
cheesecake or some reasonable facsimile thereof).
Now, will you still lose weight if you miscombine? You
might, but probably not, so don't expect to. Then
again, you probably won't gain either, unless you
REALLY misbehave—you know, really pig out. But
why would you do that? Pigging out is something you

had to do when you didn't have permission to eat something fattening. Tonight you have permission to eat anything you want and it is not considered cheating. So, since you're not cheating by eating something you shouldn't, something that you'll never be able to eat again, you don't have to eat all of it.

When you can appreciate this philosophy, adopt it and make it your own, and you learn to behave yourself, there will be plenty of next times. Tonight is just the first of the many forthcoming OWD's (opens with discretion) when you'll learn and experience, as the late great acting coach, Stella Adler, put it, "what you choose to eat determines what you have to eat."

A reminder for the future, for when you're completely on your own: Realizing that nothing successfully digests after protein except more protein, when you know you'll be eating a miscombination, never have protein in a meal preceding it. For example, don't have chicken in your salad at lunch when you plan on having a Mexican meal for dinner.

There's one more thing I'd like you to do tonight: Begin to practice my credo of making every bite count—don't waste even one. If what you've chosen to eat doesn't taste good, don't eat it. Believe me, it won't get better, so why bother? And don't be surprised when it keeps happening. You'll encounter many foods you thought were great, but then don't live up to your expectations. You see, many of our favorite foods taste better when we eat them in the closet covered with the salt of our tears and the bitter aftertaste of regret.

One of the most important parts of tonight's meal is that you'll begin to appreciate, understand and internalize my chief credo: *Think about food when it doesn't count, so you don't have to think about it when it does.* Tonight you don't have to worry, you can enjoy your meal without guilt or fear because knowing an open meal is coming up, you've already thought about what to eat. Well actually, I thought about it for you, so you're all set up for it enzymatically. So just relax and, if you feel yourself getting carried away, eating too much or just starting to get out of control, stop for a moment, take a deep breath, look at your plate and remind yourself that *it's not leaving the planet.*

 Don't forget to weigh yourself tomorrow.

DAY 15

Pineapple
Mazel Salad

Well, what did your scale say today? Did it work? Did you get away with your first open-with-discretion meal without gaining weight?

You did weigh yourself today, didn't you? What do you mean you were afraid to. Go, get on that scale right now.

How are we ever going to find out what you can get away with if you don't weigh yourself? The scale, once again, is not your judge and jury; it is your best friend. It doesn't tell you if you've been good or bad, it tells you if what you ate did or didn't work. By that I mean, did your body handle it? Did it digest what you fed it? Did the scale go down? Did you lose weight? Well, then, I guess your body needed and utilized what it was fed. It ate it up and then some more.

Did it stay the same? Bravo, that means that despite the fact that the carbohydrate portion of the meal got trapped in your stomach with the protein and didn't digest as rapidly and nutritionally as it should have, your body handled it A-okay. And obviously you didn't overeat. And you stayed in control, obviously you didn't overeat.

Don't fret if you gained weight; there are a number of factors that could have come into play. First of all, as you already know, when you mix proteins and carbohydrates, you have a mixture that just doesn't mix or digest well. If it had cheese in it, that was a double whammy. Cheese, I'm sorry to say, is a toughy. It takes hours and hours for your body to process while trapping everything else eaten along without it, further inhibiting digestion. Now, that doesn't mean you'll never be able to eat cheese. No way! I don't want to take away your enchiladas and nachos supreme, your favorite pizza or bacon-cheeseburger. Even if it does make you gain weight, you'll make it work.

You see, that's the beauty of Conscious Combining and Conscious Compensation: no matter how hard the combination is to digest, there is an antidote, an after-food, and there is a precedote (a pre-food) that will aid in its digestion. By eating these foods before and after your hard-to-digest combination, you'll aid in its digestion and not get fat.

Remember, gaining weight, by my way of thinking, is caused by food not being digested. It is simply the result of indigestion. If what you ate was broken down into nutrients the way it should have been, when it should have been, and if those nutrients, vitamins and minerals had been absorbed by your cells the way they should have been, and if the glucose had been efficiently turned into energy and the amino acids into building blocks, if your body had properly utilized what it was given and eliminated the waste, there would be nothing left over. There would be no weight gain. Somewhere along the line something got trapped. It did not get to where it needed to go, the way it should have, when it should have. Instead, it just sat there. You see, if those calories were efficiently processed, they would have turned to extra energy, not fat.

Enter your trusty pineapple, your antidote for today. The pineapple enzymes will go to work by activating the hydrochloric acid in your stomach, burning up whatever is still left. At the same time, its high levels of potassium will help reestablish your electrolyte balance to counteract any side effects of added salt. Salt, by the way, could have been the chief culprit for any gain. If your food was salty or you're just salt sensitive, your body will respond by retaining water.

Trust me, if you eat a lot of pineapple today, its high levels of potassium will help with the water retention, while its fat-burning enzymes will work hand-in-hand with your Mazel salad tonight. All that rich chlorophyll will not only help oxygenate your blood and give it an extra boost, it will also absorb some of the fat that the pineapple enzymes burned up. Additionally, the high fiber in the salad, as well as the oil in the dressing, will help clean out some of the residue of the fat the pineapple has loosened up.

If you've gained, there is one other possibility. You probably ate more than your body could efficiently handle. You overdid it. Don't worry, it's okay. It's your nature. If you could have eaten small portions, you would have. If you could have remained totally in control, and exercised willpower and discipline, and stopped when your stomach said enough while your mouth as well as your heart cried "feed me!", you would have. You'd also be thin and wouldn't need me or *The New Beverly Hills Diet* program. Perhaps the next time, you'll try eating less.

How many OWD's you can get away with depends on you: how much you eat and what you are willing to give up.

If you have gained, reassess what you ate and drank yesterday, bite for bite. Write it down on the page entitled "Rehash Sheet" (p. 102). Include every morsel, every bite, every lick of the finger. Then go over your list. Think about it: was there anything you ate that wasn't worth it, that you would be willing to give up next time? Cross it off your list. Now go over the list again, looking only at the carbohydrates. Remember, the protein portion of the meal is trapping those carbohydrates, so see if there are some you can eliminate the next time you try this same meal. Every bit of every bite makes a difference, so even giving up a little lettuce would help. *Anything* that you do in the future that's better than what you did yesterday is going to be an improvement. The next time you have an OWD meal, see what happens if you try this meal once again, minus those things you crossed out. You'll know if you are successful by the numbers on your scale.

Properly utilizing the Conscious Combining technique to arrange your diet is fun, challenging and rewarding. If you play by the rules, you can't help but win. Again, never eat fruit with anything else.

Carbohydrates go with carbohydrates. Proteins go with proteins. Fats go with either protein or carbohydrates, but not with fruit, and minimal carbs after protein. Do this religiously while we're together and forever more and you'll always stay thin.

True, you'll never gain weight if you don't miscombine—but then, where's the fun? The challenge and fun come from stretching the rules, successfully miscombining while being able to get and stay slim, and feel great.

Notice I said feel great. Remember, miscombining is not as healthy as sticking to one category. When you miscombine, much of the carbohydrate portion of the miscombination is not properly and efficiently digested. This means your body is not reaping the full nutritional value of the meal or its energy-giving potential. In fact, this extra burden you've placed on your digestive system is slowing you down.

Glorious miscombinations, however, are an integral part of our lives, and we have proved over and over that we can't live without them. And you won't have to with your scale as a guide. You are going to experiment without fear of fat and you'll see just how much you can get away with. (More than you ever dreamt was possible!)

Oh, by the way, if you did gain today, don't worry—it will come right off. The next two days will take care of it and then some. If you stayed the same or lost weight, then you're on a roll and you should see some real changes. Your body is going to shrink before your very eyes.

Quick—go run to that mirror and look at those soon-to-be-slim thighs.

D A Y   1 6

Dried Apricots
Papaya
Pineapple

Apricots provide potassium, papaya softens, pineapple burns . . .

Right now these fruits are creating your weight loss. Later they will be used to sustain your weight loss.

As you recall, yesterday I referred to antidotes and precedotes. They are listed in "Corrective Counterparts" (p. 111). Precedotes are the fruits you should eat the morning of the day of an eating experience that you know, *or think,* will be hard to digest. These fruits will set you up enzymatically and nutritionally to help make the foods you are about to eat more digestible or less fattening. The fruits you ate three days ago on your open-with-discretion day were precedotes. Antidotes are for the day after a specific type of a meal. The pineapple and the Mazel salad you ate the day after your open-with-discretion were antidotes. Notice how they are broken down into categories: before and after greasy, creamy or cheesy, specific proteins, sweets, salty foods, maxi-carb overdose, even special meals and holidays.

On page 110, you'll find "Drastic Measures After a Drastic Disaster" just in case you get crazy and go off the program. Don't say you'll never do it, and don't be too hard on yourself if and when you do. Just understand yourself and be proud of who and what you are. You're special, you know, you're an "eater," and believe me, it's nothing to be ashamed of. You don't ever need to change—your personality, that is. Your body is another story.

In developing *The New Beverly Hills Diet* program first for myself and later my clients, I have been propelled by the power of emotions. I know that our hearts are locked into our eating and any lifetime diet must include not only the foods that feed our bodies and fill our stomachs, but the foods that feed our souls and fill our hearts.

Those of us who love to eat and live to eat— "eaters"—fall into a special category: almost all of us, at one time or another, have been described as sensitive. It's always said in hushed tones, as if sensitivity is a bad thing, something of which to be ashamed. "Shh," they say, "be careful—she's sensitive." Sensitivity is about feelings. It's being alive. "Eaters" are feelers. For us, our need to eat comes not from a physical hunger but from an emotional hunger. It's our hearts that need the nourishment and our souls that need to be fed.

We swallow our disappointments, we swallow our hurt, we swallow our anger and we swallow our pride. We "eaters," we feelers, will all too often swallow our feelings because publicly and even privately it's the most acceptable way of dealing with them.

We eat when we're excited. We eat when we're sad.

We eat when we have too much to do or not enough to do. We eat when we want to escape reality or when we want to connect to it. When a nightmare wakes us in the middle of the night, food brings reality back into focus.

Eating helps us preserve our sanity. When our pain is too intense, eating soothes us—or so we think. Believe me, it doesn't. It creates a pain all its own. It only prolongs the misery. But we blot this out, obsessed only with the very real, transitory pleasure the food and the act of eating give us.

"Eaters" are sensual people, far more so than noneaters. After all, eating can only be described as a highly sensual experience. While we may not acknowledge this trait of ours, this life energy tends to frighten us. This sensuality is so intense and often so awesome that we often eat not only to satisfy our need, but also to mask it both from ourselves and from others.

"Eaters" are high-energy, creative, striving people. We eat out of frustration when our power and energy are scattered and unfocused. If we haven't found our creative avenue, we turn to food. Or we eat to "celebrate" or ease off a high, typically after an achievement, after our creativity is spent, to fill the void that comes with accomplishment, the empty space of "what's next?"

"Eaters" are "wanters." And we want what we want when we want it, and we want it all right now. "More, more, more. . . . Give me more." Too much is never enough. If something is good, more is better. The closest star is never good enough. We've got to have the star farthest away. We're never satisfied. For most of us, if we don't have what we want right now, we think the world will explode. "Eaters" are not patient people.

We are the masters of setting unrealistic goals. And we are constantly frustrated, constantly wanting.

Because eating is an emotional response to an emotional situation we get unclear messages from our bodies. Since most of us don't even know where our stomachs are, we can't hear our little cells yelling, "Feed me, nourish me, it's my turn." Instead, we respond only to the heart. Well, I'm not going to take your heart out of your stomach; I'm just going to put your head in by getting you to really think about food. You won't have to give up the one thing that makes life work for you: food. You are learning a way of eating that will allow you to be as compulsive as you need to be. I'm not going to make you change an aspect of your personality as inherent as the color of your eyes. I'm not going to make you stop eating, but I am going to make you start thinking and feeling.

As I said a couple of days ago, how you feel is based on what you eat, pure and simple. Soon your body will tell you what it needs and you'll be able to hear it. Your Skinny voice will begin to talk and you'll listen.

Soon habits will no longer dictate what you eat, nor will eating be only an emotional response to an emotional situation. No longer will hunger be like an assailant coming out of the dark, giving you a quick rabbit punch in the neck. Your heart will say go and your head will say no, and you'll begin to listen to your head. You'll continue to love to eat and live to eat, but you'll begin to eat to live. And, as you realize and experience that nothing is leaving the planet, that it will all be here tomorrow and the next day and the day after that for you to enjoy, you'll get a feeling for later. You'll begin to think about later and tomorrow and feeling good. So, in those moments of madness when all hell breaks loose and you are like a soul possessed and your heart is shouting feed me, feed me, when, with wild abandon, without discrimination, you would like to shove it in with both hands, you simply won't be able to. It will no longer work. It won't feel good.

But you'll still eat. The truth is, you'll always love to eat in those "moments of madness," and that's okay. But you'll become aware of a brief moment of clarity in the midst of "being possessed," a moment in which you have a choice. The choice does not have to be not to eat. The choice will be about not destroying yourself in the process. Food will work for you if you'll only let it.

When the need to eat is all-consuming, when your heart is shouting go and your head is shouting no, you'll listen to them both. A synergy will develop between your head and your heart, and, most important, you'll begin to choose to feel good because it feels a lot better than feeling bad. Eating and feeling good are what *The New Beverly Hills Diet* program is all about. Come on, go for it . . .

What have you got to lose?

D A Y   1 7

Watermelon

Well, it's another wash day, so be sure to eat a lot of watermelon so it can really do its job.

I hope by now you've learned to *always* take your fruit, and a lot of it, with you just in case you get hungry. If you haven't been, please do; it's important. You can't allow yourself to be a victim. What if you get hungry? Forget about hunger—what about feeling? You never know when those emotions are going to sneak up and grab you.

It's interesting to consider the ways in which we set ourselves up to fail, the ploys we use. I call them the subtle subterfuges. You know what I mean . . . preparing your favorite meal for your family on a watermelon day or bringing a sick friend your favorite chocolates. How about baking and freezing Christmas cookies in July? Or standing right next to the hors d'oeuvres table at a cocktail party? The worst one of all is trying to keep your diet a secret.

The saddest part about all this is that we don't even realize what we're doing. We aren't even aware of all the unconscious things we do to ourselves that cause us to fail. Take heart . . . this time you won't fail because I won't let you. Soon you won't let yourself, not once you recognize your own subtle subterfuges and how to avoid them.

First and foremost, you must never let yourself be a victim. Never set yourself up for failure by running out of what you need—the food you are supposed to be eating. Always buy a lot and make sure you have more than enough. If you have any left over, you can always cut it up and stick it in your freezer.

You never know when your emotions are going to sneak up and grab you, so don't leave your house for more than 12 minutes without your food. Sandwich bags, plastic containers and aluminum foil are quite wonderful inventions. Always, always, always have plenty of your food with you and be careful about sharing. Everyone will want to eat your food, especially on grape days. Don't let them. Your generosity can get you in trouble. What's going to happen if you run out?

I repeat: one of the worst things you can do is keep your diet a secret. Please, I can't stress this strongly enough, YOU MUST talk about your diet. Tell the world what you are doing. Trust me, no one will be surprised—certainly by now people have noticed. Your watermelons and papayas have not exactly been unobtrusive, but then, neither has your *thinner* body.

Getting thin requires developing a support system, a support system that is active and alive, a support system you can call your own. You can't do it alone.

None of us can; we all need some help. Yes, even you. So don't be embarrassed to ask for it! You'll only develop a Skinny voice by using it. So, if you feel yourself weakening, don't be ashamed to ask for help. Tell someone how you are feeling. Let other people help you. I still do.

Letting go of your fat image and your fat consciousness will come with time. It will come from knowing that the thin person you're becoming is here to stay because you have a way of eating that ensures it, a way of eating that allows you to turn to food (even the fattening foods you love) in your moments of madness without that food turning on you.

You can be your own worst enemy. If you expect to be perfect, to never blow it again, to only eat the so-called "safe" foods, you are setting yourself up to fail.

You love to eat, you live to eat, and it's been killing you. It is a conflict that, until *The New Beverly Hills Diet*, you haven't been able to resolve. How do you eat and stay thin?

So, you've hidden from it. You have sneaked food and you have denied your enjoyment of it in your eagerness to please yourself and those around you, and to not be rude. This constant denial of what you are has only made you what you don't want to be . . . FAT!

Why try to shut the mouth of an "eater"? Use it and embrace it. Once you've given yourself permission to eat, your love of eating won't hurt you anymore. You'll gain control.

Thin people have permission to eat happily, and so do you. It's your guilt that's working against you. Guilt is an emotion of the heart. Enjoyment is an emotion of the intellect. Your fat consciousness is overloaded with guilt, laden with regrets and "if only's" and "tomorrow's." Fat comes from the heart, thin comes from the head.

Nobody expects you to be perfect in your eating behavior—nobody, that is, except you. So stop dwelling on the negative. Just relax, and in the process of becoming a thin person, you'll learn what made you a fat person. If you do blow it, don't heap even more blame on yourself. Accentuate your positive qualities. Accentuate the times you didn't blow it, all those times you resisted the temptation.

So, you made a mistake. Big deal. Think about all the times you didn't make a mistake. Don't dwell on the negative. Stop interfering with your natural developmental process, your transformation into a Conscious Combiner and a Skinny. Stop judging yourself and expecting too much of yourself; this is going to take time. You didn't gain your weight in a day, so how can you expect to lose it in a day? If it were that easy, if there were some magic, a miracle to be had, I promise you, it would have been unearthed by now.

The only miracle there is in losing weight is finding a discipline, a way of eating you can stick to, and you have—*The New Beverly Hills Diet* program.

The magic pill hasn't been discovered. Rather, the magic is in your soul. It's in that Skinny voice of yours that is waiting to be nurtured and set free forever—and you're doing it; that's the miracle.

DAY 18

Figs
Dessert of Choice
Meat/Protein

If people haven't already started noticing your weight loss, they probably will today. As I predicted, these last three days were real winners—or should I say, losers?

In addition to all the compliments you'll be getting, another treat is in store for you today—an all-dessert meal! That's two normal-size portions of any dessert you fancy. . . . What's a normal portion? A restaurant serving portion is a good guide, but you decide for yourself when enough is enough. Remember, you don't want to gain weight, and you shouldn't for two reasons: the way the food is planned today and the discretion you'll be using . . . when you don't pig out!.

A bit of advice: unless your favorite dessert is a miscombination such as pie à la mode, try to keep all your dessert choices in the same category—all protein or all carbohydrates. They'll be easier to digest.

Desserts, as I'm sure you've noticed, are also listed in the "Food Groups" chart (p. 113).

It's not necessary to sit down and eat all or both desserts at one time. You can stretch them out over as long a period as you wish. If you aren't a dessert-eater, you can trade them in for your favorite sandwich.

Lucky for me, I've never been much of a dessert-eater. Hopefully when you start eating them in an isolated way without other foods, you, too, will begin to notice their negative side effects. Sugar (the nemesis of any dieter) is at first highly stimulating, but within a brief time has the opposite effect and causes depression and fatigue. The best way to enjoy desserts, without them enjoining you, is to eat them on their own as you are today. I can't think of anything more fattening than a trapped dessert. Just think of all those concentrated calories waiting and festering, dying to get out and become energy—instead, they turn into fat. If you do eat dessert after a meal, the only safe way to do it is to properly combine it. The food-group pages will be your savior.

It's ironic that people who complain that they are too thin are usually big sweet-eaters. The difference between you and them is that they eat sweets in place of, not after, real food. The rapid uninhibited digestion of the sugar speeds up their metabolism. It's not a very healthy way to stay thin.

Now your figs this morning can be fresh if they are in season, but nutritionally speaking, dried figs would be better (make sure they are unsulfured and no potassium sorbate has been added). Don't forget to wait at least two hours after you've eaten your last one before starting your desserts.

Tonight's meat/protein meal was selected for two reasons. If your dessert choice was a protein—ice cream, cheesecake, yogurt or one of the other protein desserts—then the protein-after-protein rule comes into play. Another equally important reason for the protein is that it will rebalance the quantity and the quality of your energy. Sugar has the potential to distort your energy as nothing else can, plus it has an addictive quality. The more you eat, the more you want, so if you don't nip it in the bud by eating something to counteract that desire, you'll get caught up on a sugar trip and you'll only want more and more and more. Red meat is the perfect counterbalance. It stops that sugar craving dead on its feet. Now, if you are not a meat-eater, then choose another protein that you do eat.

Enzymatically speaking, you'll be better off eating meat in a one-sitting-style dinner, but if you should get hungry later you can have more. And to top it all off, why not have some champagne tonight if you like to toast the fact that you've been on a diet for 18 days and haven't cheated once . . . or have you? . . . Okay, so you have.

Relax, I said it's okay, nobody expects you to be perfect, so don't be too hard on yourself. You'll change, you'll see, now that you're realizing that *if you plan for it, nothing is fattening.* And since you can plan for everything, why would you cheat . . . well you might, and since this is a probable eventuality, let's talk about how you should proceed if you do.

As you know, on the *The New Beverly Hills Diet* five-week program each day follows another for a very specific enzymatic reason: to complement, augment or embellish the processes already under way. If you should break down and cheat, do not continue with the diet as outlined. Instead, refer to "Drastic Measures After a Drastic Disaster" (p. 110). Follow the plan, taking into account the type of mistake you made and the amount of weight you gained. Once you have completed that plan, go back and pick up the diet where you left off.

Obviously, it's faster, easier and much more fun if you don't cheat.

But if you do, don't forget that the beauty of your new way of eating provides for it, and if you've blown it, there's always something you can eat that will make you feel better and lessen the blow. That's one of the miracles of this diet. It takes into account the human being in all of us.

And since you are *only human,* I repeat: Don't feel guilty. It's just a waste of time and will only perpetuate your negative fat consciousness. Besides, it's never too late to pick up where you left off even once you've blown it. It isn't the first time you have cheated and it won't be the last. So, who are we trying to kid?

We all get crazy. Remember, we "eaters" are feelers. We know that. But there is that moment of clarity when we can again begin to make conscious choices . . . to pick ourselves up, dust ourselves off and start all over again. It's easy because *The New Beverly Hills Diet* program is not like other diets. Since there are no "never's," being back on the diet doesn't mean you can never again have the foods you love, so you won't really have a good reason not to go right back on.

With your old fat consciousness, when you were on other diets and you blew it, you were never going to eat those foods you blew it with again, so you may as well cram them all in. What starts as a minor indiscretion turns into the "last supper." Three chocolate cupcakes suddenly expand into a hamburger with everything on it and a hot-fudge sundae, and before you know it, you are trying to cram a lifetime of foods into a single moment.

Since there are no never-again foods on my diet, why binge?

Oh, by the way, running out of food or not having food with them is the reason most people give for cheating. So, I repeat what I said yesterday: Always, always be prepared.

You might also be prepared with an answer when someone asks you the inevitable, "Hey, didn't you used to be fat?"

D A Y 1 9

Mango or Papaya
Pineapple
Artichokes, Asparagus or Potatoes,
Any Style

If you're getting tired of the double-fruit and all-fruit days, just be patient; I promise they won't last forever. Once you've lost your weight and you're on maintenance, you'll only need to eat fruit to start your day. You'll be able to eat regular food the rest of the time.

If you stick to carbs, then you're wide open for dinner. You can have anything except fruit. Fruit, as you know, is never eaten after anything else. After carbs you can have more carbs or you can have protein, or . . . *you can have a miscombination.*

You're not alone if you find the idea of eating all-carb meals or all-protein meals hard to grasp. See "Playing It Straight" (p. 115) for some examples. Once you understand what goes with what, you'll find these meals to be easy and enjoyable—especially the day after you've eaten a lot and you haven't gained an ounce.

Ideally, you should avoid miscombinations whenever possible. If you play it straight, if you play by the rules of combining, you'll never gain weight.

Avoiding miscombinations isn't as unappetizing as it might seem. Tonight's dinner certainly doesn't sound like a diet meal: artichokes dipped in butter, mayo or Mazel dressing; asparagus; and potatoes, any style (baked, hashed, mashed, French-fried). So, eat mangoes or papayas until you get bored, wait an hour before switching to pineapple, then wait two hours before beginning your open-carb dinner. As I said, sticking to the categories and not miscombining can still be fun, either at home, in a restaurant, or even at a champagne buffet.

Home is certainly the easiest place to practice proper combining. You're in total control and, believe me, there are untold combinations in either category that will be as tantalizing and satisfying as many of those miscombinations you love so much. Not that you have to give them up, but you just won't be able to have them all the time. You can't keep eating the way you were eating or you'll continue to look the way you were looking. Obviously, you have to give up something. Although you aren't giving up miscombining, you are going to be doing it with discretion. You are going to be picking and choosing your occasions, and the rest of the time you are going to be Consciously Combining. You are going to be thinking about food when it doesn't count so you don't have to think about it when it does.

I'm sure by now you probably have some questions. Hopefully they'll all be answered within these 35 days. If you're impatient and don't want to wait, don't hesitate to write me at my ClubSlim

Headquarters, 505 First Avenue North, Seattle, WA 98109, or visit my website and ask me there: http://www.cyberskinny.com.

Perhaps your question is one that is most frequently asked.

Q. I've just had surgery. Can I continue eating this way?

A. Consult your doctor, but I can't imagine him objecting.

Q. I've just found out I'm pregnant. Do I have to change my diet?

A. Once again, consult your doctor. Remember, your nutritional needs change and your doctor is your authority.

Q. How nutritious is it to make a meal out of doughnuts or cheesecake rather than eating it as a dessert?

A. It's not nutritious either way, but if you have it with other foods, it will get trapped. When you eat it alone it will not.

Q. Do you ever gain weight, Judy?

A. Sure, my weight fluctuates like everyone else's, and sometimes I even eat foods I know will cause me to gain weight, but I know that eating fruit in the morning will digest and eliminate those unwanted pounds.

Q. Don't you ever miss having a real meal?

A. No, I have them as often as I want, and so can you because if you follow the rules you have been learning, those "real meals" won't make you fat.

Q. What do I do if I gain my weight back again?

A. You won't—unless, of course, you disavow every rule and throw all caution to the wind. If you do, however, just pick yourself up, dust yourself off, stand naked in front of the mirror and pull out this book and start at Day 1.

D A Y 2 0

Kiwi
Open with Discretion
Protein

Today is a big test. . . . Have I been a good teacher? How much have you learned about Conscious Combining, and about yourself?

If you did not do so well on your last open day, don't worry; you'll do better this time. Experience is the best teacher. Trust me, you're developing a new consciousness and today will prove it. You've learned from your mistakes. Now that you can eat *anything,* you'll find you don't have to eat *everything.* Watch, you'll see. Today you'll really start making choices. But no matter what happens weight-wise, it will be taken care of. I've scheduled your next few days to accommodate anything that happens today, so let's see how you handle yourself and we'll go from there.

It should be clear as to why you're scheduled for a protein dinner after your open lunch—the protein rule: Once you've eaten protein, your next meal must be protein, or at least mostly protein.

219

For those of you who weighed the same or less after your first OWD, this should be especially fun. Now your Skinny self can really take control. Listen to your little Skinny voice today as it shouts down the voice of fat. Today is a very important day, so select one of your favorites for lunch, something you never give yourself permission to eat except when you get crazy. I know I've said this before, but it bears repeating. There's more to eating than meets the mouth, and more to food as it meets the stomach. You become a thin person by becoming a thin person; by confronting, acknowledging and letting go of the fat person. Well, "fat person," it's time to stop perpetuating the fat consciousness through deprivation.

Deprivation is the main reason you have always broken your diets in the past and why you have always regained your lost weight. When you live in an unreality, depriving yourself of your favorite foods, you grow more and more diet-conscious and resentful. Your favorite foods are the exceptions, but instead of allowing them to be exceptional, instead of consuming them with pleasure, you allow them to consume you with pain. By never allowing yourself to enjoy them, by never giving yourself permission to eat them openly and blissfully, you revert to them illicitly and use them as an emotional stopgap, eating them when you can least enjoy them. As I said before, "eaters" are feelers, and eating helps us stop feeling. When we eat because we're feeling, we aren't tasting. Unless, of course, it's the bitter aftertaste of guilt and recrimination at having blown our diets.

Of course you're not expected to stop eating during an emotional moment, but if you follow the rules of

Conscious Combining and stick to one category, it won't hurt you.

The trick is to stop turning your "pleasure givers" into pain relievers . . . to stop turning to your favorites when you are so caught up in emotions you can't even taste them, when it doesn't really matter what you're eating as long as you're eating, when anything that tastes good will do, when all you need to do is just swallow your feelings and dilute the emotions of the moment. Now when you think about your mother-in-law or the crises at work or your divorce or the spilled garbage, you won't turn to ice cream.

You can have your favorite foods in the clear light of day with permission and without fear. By removing the guilt, you're making your favorite foods pleasure givers instead of pain relievers. But be prepared for some surprises. You'll probably find that once you are eating with your mind as well as your heart, you won't like the way a lot of your special favorites taste or make you feel. And even more surprising is that when you allow yourself to experience the emotional moment devoid of the food that always distracted you from it, the moment will gain clarity. When you can truly experience the moment and the emotion, you'll also experience the food.

So, enjoy your lunch and your new life in the slim lane.

DAY 21

Pineapple
Two Bananas

I'm an "eater," pure and simple, and I'm proud to admit it. I've accepted it. I've acknowledged it and I've embraced it. I've surrendered, I've given up, I've given in to thin, I've let food and eating become a positive. I've learned how to make them work for me, and so can you.

I'm thin, but only because I have my technique of Conscious Combining. I'm not one of those natural skinnies who can eat everything and never gain weight. They don't think about food the way I do, they don't care about food the way I do. Food isn't important to them the way it is to me . . . and the way it is to you. Food doesn't have to make us fat. I promise you, if you follow the techniques of *The New Beverly Hills Diet* program; if you firmly integrate this new consciousness into your soul; if you truly believe that if you don't have it now, you can have it later, and if not later, then tomorrow because nothing is leaving the planet, you'll lose weight and keep it off.

When you truly believe that eating is no longer a now-or-never event, when you realize you have permission to have French fries any time you want them, not only when you're depressed, you'll become a Born-Again Skinny.

You've come a long way in just 21 days (21, the age of reason). And with each day that passes, Conscious Combining and slimhood are becoming a more deeply imbedded part of your life. It happened to me and it will happen to you. You're well on your way to getting there, and I think you know that now.

P.S. Why not try baking your bananas tonight—you'll love them. . . . Just like you're loving the new you.

DAY 22

Grapes or Cherries
A Special Bedtime Treat

Today you can have your pick of grapes or cherries, and if chocolate candies or cookies are your thing, have two or three at bedtime.

Did you say your scale has been a little crazy . . . up one day, down the next? Don't worry. It happens. I know it's frustrating, but that's the way it is and it's just another instance when a scale comes in handy. It makes us confront our frustration and deal with it without eating.

I know I've talked a lot about "eaters" and feelings. Think about all the times you swallowed your frustration or your sadness or your anger by eating. Will you ever stop eating out of response to feelings? Will food ever stop being love or comfort? Will you ever be like one of those naturally skinny people who say they're full when half the food is still on their plates, or, better yet, the skinnies that pack it away and brag about how they just can't gain an ounce? Probably not. As I said yesterday, we're not like them.

Let's take a closer look at naturally skinny people. They come in several varieties. Take the skinnies who can pack it away, for instance. They might eat a lot at one sitting, but that's it. They're meal-eaters, and they rarely take a between-meals sip of this or a nibble of that. You wouldn't catch them eating a piece of hard candy at the dry cleaners or having a frozen yogurt at 4:00 in the afternoon. They eat three meals a day and that's it. Can you do that?

Then there are the skinnies that stop after a few bites and say they're full. Don't envy them, pity them. Think of what they're missing out on. When food is in their mouths, their hearts don't sing and their souls don't soar. Their mouth is not like an "eater's" mouth. The mouth of an "eater" is like the keys of a finely tuned piano. Each bite rings out a different note, and we're only happy when they are playing in harmony. The music goes on and on, the melody is endless. But the down side to this rhapsody is that as long as the song is playing, as long as you continue to eat a variety of foods, as long as there is food in your mouth, your stomach doesn't know when it's had enough. When the mouth is on, the stomach is off.

I, like most "eaters," have an amazing capacity. As long as it tastes good, I'll keep eating. When my stomach is full, I'm usually not even aware of it. The excitement of the different tastes and textures in my mouth overrides any message my stomach may be sending to me. As far as I'm concerned, one of the greatest joys in the world is sitting around a table with family or friends eating and talking, eating and laughing, eating and planning, eating, eating, eating. As long as the food is there, I'll keep eating it.

It's amazing what happens when the stomach has had too much. When it has had more than it can handle, the body just stretches to accommodate it. Well, perhaps that's a bit simplified, but what do you think getting fat is all about?

When I first developed my style of eating, Conscious Combining, I discovered that the benefits of the Mono-Meal (one food only) were as dramatic psychologically as they were physiologically. I learned when enough was enough. While it didn't exactly transform me into a little eater, it did show me how to stop before I did any damage, how not to eat more than my body could handle. In other words, I learned how to eat as much as I could without gaining an ounce.

When you are eating only one thing at a time, sooner or later it stops tasting good. No matter how fast my heart beats on the first bite, no matter how violently my taste buds palpitate with that first swallow, sooner or later even a white chocolate truffle stops tasting good. Sooner or later the taste buds get bored and even the most orgasmic taste treat will cease to be a thrill.

Ideally it would be a lot better if my stomach said "enough" instead of my mouth, but it doesn't—at least not without a struggle. Quite frankly, I'm tired of fighting. I spent the first 29 years of my life dealing with this compulsive aspect of my personality, the part of me that says if something is good, more is better, and too much is not enough.

Now, instead of fighting it, I'm accepting it. I'm living with it and I'm making it work for me. I eat to my heart's content and I never eat my heart out. I can satisfy my need to feel really full. I never go hungry and I never feel deprived. Conscious Combining and, most particularly, the Mono-Meal, have been my salvation. They have allowed eating to bring its full potential of joy into my life.

Now, what I'm going to ask you to do is a triple whammy. First, you'll become sensitized to taste. You'll learn just how pregnant with feeling your taste buds are. Second, you'll acknowledge your stomach. You'll experience when enough is enough. And third, **you'll give up the struggle!**

On your next open meal, schedule yourself for just one specific food that means more to you than life itself, be it a chocolate soufflé, barbecued spareribs, roast duckling or Maui potato chips. Arrange an appropriate setting so that you can eat your choice openly and wantonly, without guilt, without fear, with sheer pleasure and permission. Important . . . make sure you have much more than you think you'll want or would even dream of eating. That way you won't worry about not having enough.

The idea is not to see how much you can get in, in how short a time, but how long you can make the pleasure last.

First experience the texture, the taste, the smell, how you feel and how it feels. Be aware of how that favorite food feels when it first hits your mouth, how your taste buds perk up and what happens to your tongue. Then experience your food fantasy bite for bite, slowly and luxuriously. Tune in to your stomach and try to identify the moment just before you're full. Tune in to your response and be aware. As you begin to get full, you'll notice the food will no longer taste as wonderful as it did at first bite. The more full you become, the less exciting the taste.

The first time you do this exercise, you'll probably find that you've out-eaten your stomach. But don't worry, I'm sure no damage will be done. On the contrary, you learn by doing. How will you ever know when enough is enough if you don't experience it and stop while you have the choice?

Repeat this exercise at least three times with different foods. Then, one by one, try it with all your favorites. Before you know it, every eating experience will be soul-soaring. You'll understand how food makes you feel, you'll react to being full, and overeating will be a trauma of the past. You've made the choice never to be fat again. So just enjoy your day and your reflection in the mirror.

P.S. Your Skinny is showing!

DAY 23

Prunes
Sandwich of Choice
Fisherman's Platter/Protein

Have you decided what kind of a sandwich you're going to have? How about corned beef on rye, tuna on whole wheat, or a roasted pepper, grilled onion, tomato and mushroom sandwich? How about a bacon-cheeseburger with all the fixin's? It's important that today's choice is the sandwich of your dreams at the place of your dreams; nothing less will do. Why do you think I gave you that tasting exercise yesterday for your next open meal? I knew today was coming up, I planned it. So, just relax and enjoy it . . . the eating and the exercise.

Now about tonight . . . you're probably asking yourself, "What's a fisherman's platter?"

Well, that's up to you. You can have three different kinds of fish cooked any way you prefer. Broiled lobster, oysters on the half-shell, fried shrimp, broiled halibut . . . I could go on but you get the message. If fish and chips are your thing, forget the chips (no carbs after a lunch that includes protein), but the fried fish (batter and all) is A-okay.

Again, if you have trouble deciding when enough is enough and need a little help exercising quantity control, just keep reminding yourself that you can have whatever it is you are overeating another time. *It's not leaving the planet.* Better yet, instead of depending on yourself, why not take someone with you? Actually, why not take three someones with you, but not all at once.

The time has come to prove yourself worthy of being called a "Skinny." A Skinny can eat, enjoy and not overindulge. Not once, not twice, but often and consistently, without gaining an ounce. Let's see how you do—you've got three chances.

The first time, select a "natural Skinny" for your eating partner, someone who eats a moderate amount and leaves food on his or her plate, and match him or her bite for bite, no more, no less.

For the second outing, eat with someone who has a fat consciousness, someone whose only concept of tomorrow is making tonight the last supper. Eat side by side with the overeater and prove you are a true Beverly Hills Dieter, a true Skinny. Prove it by not following his or her lead. Let him or her pig out while you don't. Try to remember and re-create what it was like when you ate with the natural Skinny.

Now for the third outing (this could be the toughest), eat with someone who is thin, but who eats like a fat person. We all know and envy this type of person, the kind who pack it away, brag about how much they can eat and never gain weight. The kind who out-ate us even in our old fat days, the ones about whom we always said, "Well, if they can do it, so can I." And you tried, only they stayed thin and you got fatter. Remember, you can't match them bite for bite, so don't even try. Just do your own thing. Again, think back to the natural Skinny. Then, with one hand hold on to your fork and with the other hand hold on to those now-prominent hipbones—and just eat like a human being.

This is only the beginning. In fact, let's call it "the first supper" because if you can repeatedly make it through these tests, then you have succeeded in cultivating your little Skinny voice to its maximum and you will **never** be fat again.

D A Y 2 4

Pineapple
Papaya
Pineapple

Well, Rome wasn't built in a day, and you won't get thin overnight. If you were trapped by something salty or ate your way into oblivion yesterday, don't worry, tomorrow is another day. I repeat, nobody expects you to be perfect. If you were perfect, then you wouldn't need *The New Beverly Hills Diet* program. I just hope that some of this is sinking in, that you are not still eating with wild abandon and stuck in that "pig out" mentality. You aren't, are you? I didn't think so!

Sooner or later you'll get it. If you didn't have it in you, you wouldn't have been able to stick with me and with this diet for this long.

Now let's hear it for those of you who ate to your hearts' content yesterday and aren't eating your heart out today. Your weight is either the same or you lost. You deserve a round of applause! I bet you can hardly hear your fat voice anymore. A word of caution: Don't get too sure of yourself or you'll really get in trouble. Turn a deaf ear to that old fat voice that says, "Now that I'm thin, I can eat anything I want to." You can't, so don't even try.

The question I'm most frequently asked is, "When I go back to eating 'normally,' will I gain all my weight back?" My answer is, "If you go back to eating the way you used to eat, then you will look just like you used to look!" Sorry to disillusion you, but you must always remember from whence you came. Even when you become thin, which you will, and even if you stay thin, which you will, you will always be a fat person because, unfortunately, those fat cells won't ever go away. They just shrink up and hang out, lying in wait to plump up again at the slightest provocation.

Believe me, staying thin is harder than getting thin because you lose the impetus. Once you're thin, your body won't embarrass you or let you down. You won't have the constant reminder of that obvious fat for the world to see. Plus, any support and encouragement you received has stopped with time and results. Now instead everyone says, "Come on, look at you, you don't have to be on a diet anymore. You're so skinny." As if you're not the person you once were, as if all those little fat cells weren't poised and ready to plump back up at a moment's notice.

A funny thing happens to all of us when we first lose weight. We play this game of "I can eat whatever I want. I'm thin now. I don't have to give food or eating a second thought." The problem is, you do have to give it a second, and a third, thought, and that's what sets you apart from the natural skinnies. You think about food a lot. If this isn't your first diet, it's because each time you've lost weight you thought,

"This time I can get away with it," and you returned, at least for the most part, to your old way of eating. Well you can't get away with it. Your old way of eating didn't work; that's why you were fat. So forget about it. Surrender, give up and give in to "thin." I have—so big deal. What's so terrible about not mis-combining foods? My favorite lunch at Nat 'n' Al's Deli in Beverly Hills of potato pancakes and French fries with coleslaw and rye bread and butter isn't exactly what you'd call deprivation!

Sure, it's tempting to eat the way non-"eaters" do. In the beginning, you have to always be on your toes, to constantly remember that fat person lurking inside you and turn a deaf ear to your well-meaning friends waving the fork of temptation and egging you on. Trust me, many of these friends are acting out of jealousy. The fat ones only wish they had your strength and the thin ones don't want you as compe-tition. So today, unless it's pineapple and papaya, take a pass.

DAY 25

Watermelon

Although no two bodies handle food in exactly the same way, the basic physical laws that govern the human body are the same for everyone. As I said earlier, every time you miscombine you will not gain weight. If that were the case, you'd weigh a ton.

How will you maintain your new weight? How do you figure out how much you can get away with, without gaining back your lost weight? Each person's capacity to stretch the rules of Conscious Combining is different. The most important factor is your relationship to food and the role it plays in your life.

The more important food is to you, the more it usurps your energy and your power, the less you can get away with. I, for example, get by with very few transgressions. But those of you who fit into the "social fat" category and aren't emotionally attached to food will be able to get away with a lot more than the rest of us.

Maintaining your weight means experimenting without fear. The worst that can happen is you'll gain a pound or two. That's a necessary part of your learning process. You'll find some foods will be harder for your body to digest than others. Maintenance is all about seeing what works and what doesn't work for you as an individual. This is your diet. You're taking my rules and creating a diet, a way of life for yourself—forever.

If something doesn't work, if you gain weight when you eat it, if it turns out to be "fattening," you are going to learn how to make it work. You'll learn how to make it less fattening by counteracting or negating its negative side effects—the extra pounds on your scale. That's what separates *The New Beverly Hills Diet* program from all the other diets. You won't have to give up the things that don't work—the things that make you gain weight—because you'll make them work. That's what you're learning to do. That's what Conscious Combining and Conscious Compensation are all about.

I hope that by now you've exposed your little secret to the world. I'm sure that everyone who knows you has spotted the difference and knows why, and most of them have been willing to overlook your little idiosyncrasies (like toting your own pineapple to dinner). They like the new thin you. For those of you who haven't gone public, it's time to flaunt those hipbones and have a fruit meal outside your house. Since today is a watermelon day, it is a watermelon meal. A word of reassurance: Once you're on maintenance, the all-fruit days will be far less frequent than when you are trying to lose, but those days are a reality, so you'd better stay in shape literally as well as figuratively.

The only way you'll make this way of eating your own is by integrating it into your everyday life. Think about it. How many times did you eat outside your house last week or the week before? Or if you didn't because your diet stopped you, think about how many times you would have if you weren't on a diet. I'm sure it's been easy at home, in an environment that you can control, but the tough part is the out-side world. That's where you really use all those excuses and exceptions you're so good at: the parties, the dinners, the business lunches, the galas, the ball games, the picnics, the trips, the birthdays and the vacations, especially the vacations. The reality is, our lives are filled with exceptions and if we only "watch it" at home, thin will always be a never.

So now it's time to take your newfound knowledge along with your newfound friends—your watermelon and your hipbones—and go public. I mean that lit-erally. Don't you think it's about time you bragged a little? *You used to be fat, you're not fat anymore, and you will never be fat again!* So if you haven't already shouted your success from the rooftops, what better day to do it than on a watermelon day? That goes for all of you, even those of you who still have pounds to lose.

The whole idea of this exercise is to break the con-ventional cycle of simply taking what comes our way. We make conscious choices in every other part of our lives, but it's as if we forget that we can make a choice about our bodies. The feeding and care of our bodies can be selective, not reactive. In truth, we are a food-oriented society. We socialize with food. We do business over food. We celebrate with food. One-upmanship these days seems to ride on out-cooking one another. Cooking and eating are our number one national pastime. Obviously in these first few weeks of the diet, you've had to make a few social adjustments. Eventually, however, you'll be able to schedule your eating orgies to take full advantage of your social calendar.

The exercises you've been doing—taking your watermelon public or eating with three different eaters—will have changed your consciousness so that you'll never again have to be a victim of every social experience. Always remind yourself that nothing is leaving the planet. It will all be there tomorrow, and tomorrow means a choice, the choice to be thin.

What you forgo today, you can fill up on tomorrow.

DAY 26

On Your Own

Tomorrow is here and it's here for you to enjoy. Now you're ready to begin living and making choices based on eating what you really want, not what you *think* you should want or *think* you should have. But then, you made the biggest choice of all: *the choice to be thin.* These next two days are very special; they will mark that transition from temporary to forever.

I suppose you could throw caution to the wind and consider these two days license to go mad and eat everything, but why would you do that when you can eat everything anyhow? Remember, you're not on a diet. Conscious Combining isn't a jail sentence or something you have to do. It's a way of life, your miracle line to happiness and "forever thin." It's something you do for yourself, your body, your sense of well-being, your head and your soul. You are gaining control. You're letting go of the fat consciousness that screams "feed me, feed me!" That voice no longer dominates your world. It is no longer the last voice you hear when you go to sleep at night and the first voice you hear in the morning. Fat is no longer crowding out your world. Your energy and your power are your own. You are free. You are no longer your own worst enemy. The old diet consciousness— the anxieties and insecurities caused by being fat, hating yourself, never enjoying the food you were inhaling—is vanishing. Isn't it wonderful not to be ashamed of eating anymore? Not to be ashamed of yourself? Now it's time to prove it, to really make this way of eating your own. Sooner or later you've got to start thinking and doing for yourself. Lock into a world where you can participate and partake in all the "good's" the good life has to offer, including whatever you want to eat and a body of which you can be proud, a world where you will soon see that you can be as thin as you'd like for the rest of your life while having your cake and eating it, too.

These next two days are not license to go hog wild and gain weight, but I also don't want you to perpetuate the deprivation drag and make these all-fruit days or heavy-duty weight-loss days. Every day of your life is not a weight-loss day. Every day of your life isn't about being on your diet and losing, or being off your diet and gaining. How about just "being." That's precisely what you are going to do for the next two days. You are going to take a break, go off the rigid regimen of weight loss and move into the wonderful wide-open world of maintenance. It's an opportunity to prove to your Skinny self what I've just said. Remember, life isn't just about being on a diet or off a diet, and every day of your life does not have to be a weight-loss day. I just want you to see how much you can get away with and stay the same.

How much that will be, will depend on you. Each person's capacity to stretch the limits is different. The more important food is to you, the less you can get away with.

Now, let's talk about what you're going to eat today. . . . If you long for your old familiar breakfast or perhaps your "fantasy" breakfast, then go for it, but with one hand and one bite at a time.

You'll be way ahead of the game if you start the day with the appropriate fruit. That's where the precedotes come in, the fruits that will enzymatically set you up for the other foods you'll be eating today. Remember, though, it's two hours before you can eat again, so plan accordingly and get up extra early. If, however, you haven't risen early enough and there really isn't enough time to eat fruit and wait two hours, then make this one of the rare days you don't start with fruit. Make your on-your-own breakfast your first eating experience of the day.

As you already know, **what you choose to eat determines what you have to eat,** so if there is protein in that breakfast, you're locked into 80 percent protein for the balance of the day. Ideally, it should be all-protein for the rest of the day because, as you already know, once protein has been introduced into your stomach no carbohydrates can efficiently digest that same day. In my original *The Beverly Hills Diet* I was rigid about that rule: Once you had eaten protein in the course of the day, you had to stick with protein; nary a carbohydrate could pass those lips, or slip down that throat. Well, time, experience and experiments have shown that most people can stretch this rule if they limit the carbohydrates they eat after their first mixed meal. By limit, I mean at least 80 percent of any meal following should then be protein. More than that or, heaven forbid, a meal consisting predominantly of carbohydrates after a protein meal is really playing with fire, or should I say, fat.

If your miscombination is at lunch, you'll follow the protein rule for your dinner or any snacking you might do in between.

That's right, snacking today is perfectly fine as long as you stick to your categories and wait the appropriate time.

I hope that, by now, you've stopped thinking of eating in the traditional mealtimes of breakfast, lunch and dinner, and started practicing eating as food experiences separated by one- and two-hour increments. If you have, this will ensure that your new Skinny self will take hold and stay forever.

Before you go to sleep tonight, spend a few minutes rehashing what you ate today and record it on the "Rehash Sheet" in "The Born Again Skinny Diary" (p. 102). Then pat yourself on the back for what a good little Skinny you are.

D A Y 2 7

On Your Own

Even though you're still on your own, you **must** start today with fruit—either as an antidote because your weight is up, or as a precedote if your weight stayed the same (see "Corrective Counterparts," p. 111). I won't even ask if you've weighed yourself today. I know you have. At this point I'm sure you have glorified and solidified your love affair with your scale; it should be as important to you as food. It isn't rewarding or punishing you. It merely tells you what does or doesn't work. It is your single most important tool for achieving eternal slimhood.

The one exception to those starting today with fruit would be those whose weight was down today and who started with fruit yesterday. You may want to see how well your body and your energy handle a day with no fruit, just be sure, however, to follow the other rules for the rest of the day.

Some of you may be saying, "But wait, I didn't start with fruit yesterday and my weight didn't go up. Why can't I do it again today?" You could, but you'd be taking a chance. Is it really worth it? You now know that starting your days with fruit is the key to keeping you thin forever. While you can get away with an occasional "off day" (I do mean occasional, not more than one a week), I don't want you to get into the bad habit of tampering with the foundation, lest the structure crumble and those mountains of flesh return.

Now that you are plugged into the potency of fruit to get and keep you thin, you must make that rule a priority. Put it along with the other Golden Rules on a high pedestal and internalize them so that they always guide your eating. Make them as much a part of your life, as much a part of your daily code of behavior, as the Ten Commandments. Make a commitment to me and to yourself to establish these few simple parameters:

Golden Rule #1—Weigh yourself *every* day.

Golden Rule #2 (fruit)—Start almost every day of your life with fruit. Once you have eaten something other than fruit in the course of the day, do not eat fruit again that day.

Remember, fruit digests almost instantly. Before you can even finish eating a pineapple, its nutrients are being absorbed by your body. If it is inhibited in its digestion, if it is eaten after anything else, it gets trapped in your stomach by other foods. Its explosive enzyme action will be offset by bloating and gas. Your savior will be transformed into your tormentor.

Golden Rule #3 (the waiting time)—When you go from fruit to fruit, wait one hour. When you go from one food group to another, wait two hours minimum (three would be better).

These are the minimum waiting times—the shortest periods of time you can get away with, without running the risk of fat. Remember, you gain weight because food is not processed properly. In simpler terms, if food doesn't leave your stomach when it should, if it becomes trapped or held up by other antagonistic foods, the nutrients it should generate will not be properly processed by your body and you'll gain weight.

Golden Rule #4 (protein)—Once you've eaten protein, eat at least 80 percent protein for the remainder of the day. (The "Golden Rules" are listed for easy reference on p. 104.)

Of course, nothing is carved in stone. There are many variables. Following these four rules, however, will make the difference between thin and fat, life and lifeless, happiness and misery, temporarily and FOREVER THIN.

DAY 28

Pineapple
Papaya
Pineapple

You want to believe, but you're tentative. How many times have you heard the promise of "forever"? You think it's too good to be true. You've heard so many vacant promises. You've believed, but again and again your belief was battered and denied. I don't blame you for being a skeptic. Statistically the odds are 9 to 1 against keeping off pounds lost on a traditional diet, a diet that *excluded* your favorite foods. I don't blame you for being terrified, the statistics are devastating. But trust me and trust your scale. The past two days should have put those fears to rest. If you behaved yourself, I'm sure you're hugging your scale, reveling in your hipbones, locking in to *The New Beverly Hills Diet* program. You're now in control. Have you noticed that when you control your eating, the rest of the world falls into line, that now your power is no longer scattered and diffused . . . you are no longer consumed with thoughts of food, but rather with thoughts of staying thin and feeling

251

good? Well, here are some tools that will help perpetuate those thoughts.

1. *First and foremost, experience and enjoy.* Remember, it's not how much you can eat in how
   short a time, it's how long you can make the
   pleasure last. You have permission to experience and enjoy, so eat slowly. Luxuriate in the
   taste and understand how it makes you feel.

2. *Ease into maintenance.* When you begin maintenance and resume "regular eating," do it gently
   and always be prepared for the worst. It takes a
   full six months of maintenance before your body
   is truly in balance at your new weight . . . before
   your heart is in harmony with your new way of
   eating.

3. *Isolate your eating experiences so that you can
   isolate their effects.* Know your enemy so that
   you'll know how to defend yourself. This is a very
   important tool. It is the keystone to learning to
   stretch the rules. If you find that you gain weight
   from a particular eating experience, it's not the
   end of the world. On the contrary, that's how
   you'll learn to correct it. Repeat your experiments. Often those most devastating in the early
   stages of maintenance (particularly salt) will be
   quite successful after your body has had more
   time to stabilize—after the first six months.

4. *Experiment—stretch every rule to its limit.* Don't
   be afraid. Only in this way can you identify the
   parameters of your Skinny kingdom. If you don't
   know for sure just how far you can go, you'll
   never be able to stay where you are. Find out

what works for you and what doesn't. After all, we're talking about forever. Try café au lait at the end of a protein day. See how many open meals you can manage in a week. Find out what happens if you eat as much as you want of your favorite pizza, how it feels to be buried under mounds of mozzarella. Eat pancakes until you turn into the Pillsbury Doughboy.

Juggle your combos of precedotes and antidotes and learn what works best for you and when. Relish your control. Play with those enzymes until you know every nuance and every possibility. Take control once and for all. Don't cower in the safety zone. You have nothing to be afraid of. There is no damage you can't correct, no pounds gained that you can't lose. You're on *The New Beverly Hills Diet* program and that's forever. You're skinny now and will be forever.

5. *Don't deprive yourself.* Schedule in your favorite foods and eat them with wild abandon. They are the exceptions, so make them exceptional. Consume them, or they will consume you. If you don't schedule them in, you are setting yourself up for failure. If you turned to ice cream when your mother yelled at you, if you buried yourself in barbecued spareribs when a romance soured, if you turned to chocolate to blot out a bad day, be alert! If you're not careful these foods will continue to be your refuge. You'll continue to indulge yourself with them in emotional moments. But in the clear light of day, if you schedule them in unsullied by feeling and with permission, if you allow yourself to experience

them unemotionally and happily without guilt, you'll win the battle of the binge. You'll not only diffuse the emotion of food, you may even find out that, unmasked by emotion, many of the foods you thought were so terrific really aren't. Somehow they lose their flavor when they aren't covered with salty tears.

If you can't eat your favorite foods when you're perfect, when can you, and then what's the point? In your devious little mind, you'll still be on a diet that means deprivation, a diet that you have to "cheat on." You'll have opened the door for your fat consciousness to move in and crowd out your Skinny soul. If you don't schedule in your favorite foods, you're denying the heart of *The New Beverly Hills Diet* program and you're not making it your own. Remember, this eating plan focuses on what you want to eat, and that determines what you *have* to eat. So stop denying yourself. You deserve to have what you really want. You've earned it!

DAY 29

Watermelon or Grapes

Neither one of these fruit days is new to you and by now you should know which one works better. "Works better" not only means affects more of a weight loss, but also refers to how it makes you feel. Remember, this is as much about feeling good as it is about keeping off the weight you've already lost and the weight you will continue to lose.

For those who still have a way to go and will not finish their weight-loss regimen by Day 35—don't worry. I'll be getting back to you. Right now I'd like to continue talking about "maintenance."

Your first six months as a Skinny are crucial; your fat is on hold, ready to pounce back at the slightest sliver of opportunity. It doesn't need much provocation. It's in the beginning when you are newly thin that you are at your most vulnerable, physically and psychologically. Physically, although gorgeous and radiantly thin, your body is unstable and still dangerously prone to fat. Remember, those fat cells haven't gone away, and in the beginning, particularly, they just lie in wait, waiting to be fed and to plump back up again. Mentally, you are subject to alternating states of happiness and complacency and the "just one bite won't hurt" mentality. Your fat consciousness is primed for action and will take mental advantage in an instant. Unless this is the first time you've ever lost weight, it has always made a comeback before and it's lying in wait, coiled to strike.

Plan on taking a good six months to acclimate your body and your brain to your new lifestyle—*The New Beverly Hills Diet* program—and to make Conscious Combining unconscious.

First and foremost, weigh yourself every day for the first six months. Write it down. When you travel, take your scale with you. Perpetuate that love affair, your scale is your only impartial observer of your perfection.

Midnight does not a new day make. A day ends when you go to sleep, and the new one begins when you wake up, not when the clock strikes 12. If you awaken hungry in the middle of the night, continue eating the last thing you ate before you went to sleep.

Always remember that you lost weight by feeding your body, not by starving it. Eating will also keep you thin. It's eating the proper foods before and after miscombinations that will make them work and keep them from being fattening.

- When you're in doubt, and you don't know what corrective counterpart to use, eat pineapple, it's the closest thing to a miracle food that there is.

Don't overdo it, though. If you eat it too often, its effectiveness will diminish dramatically.

- Neutral fruits can be eaten any time you don't need a corrective counterpart. They can also be used as a precedote to an open-with-discretion meal. Enjoy them and take advantage of them. They make a welcome change from our trusty enzymatics.
- Fruit should start roughly 90 percent of your mornings. Fruit clears you out from the day before and sets you up for whatever foods you'll be eating later. Unless you need a specific precedote, virtually any fruit qualifies, and that includes the neutrals, such as peaches, pears, nectarines and apricots.
- As a general rule, dried fruits should not be eaten the meal before or for breakfast the morning following an animal protein. It tends to cause gas.
- Don't begin the day with raisins or dates. They are too concentrated, too intense.
- Nuts and seeds should always be raw and unsalted—unsalted for obvious reasons and raw for the lecithin your body needs.
- I hope you've learned to love your coffee or tea black. Remember the protein rule: a drop of milk in your morning coffee or your afternoon tea can be far more devastating than a pound of chocolates. If you still miss it, try adding cinnamon to the grounds before brewing, or use Rice Dream as I mentioned earlier.
- Plan your menus a week at a time. Schedule in your emotional, as well as your social and business, needs.

Be generous and imaginative! What you choose to eat determines what you have to eat. It's your life, it's your diet and it's your agenda. Remember, once you're on maintenance, you aren't on a "diet." You aren't trying to lose weight. Deprivation only breeds overindulgence. Enjoy food, enjoy eating, enjoy cooking, and enjoy entertaining. Enjoy and start living!

- When preparing for a meal, keep yourself "enzymatically open." When you know that later on in a given day you'll be eating a miscombination, a fruit precedote is ideal. Don't avoid eating. "Starving yourself" is just a perpetuation of your fat consciousness. Not only will you be ravenous when the time comes to eat, but your body, suddenly inundated by a barrage of food, will simply not be able to function efficiently. Consider how long it takes a garbage disposal to start working when you first turn it on.

- As a general practice, maxi-carbs should not be eaten the meal before or the meal after protein. Don't, for example, have bagels for breakfast and chicken and ribs for lunch, lamb for dinner and pancakes for breakfast. You'll be able to get away with it occasionally, but not as a daily practice.

Ideally, an all-protein day should be divided into only three eating experiences. Try to keep nibbling to a minimum. Each protein meal should be separated by at least six hours.

A word of caution: If you are on only protein, you can selectively eat only the protein from a dish that mixes protein and carbohydrates, but you cannot do the opposite. That is, you cannot pick out and eat the carbohydrates and leave the protein. Take a chicken and rice casserole, for example. If you're on protein, you can safely pick out and eat the chicken, but if you're on carbs and think you can get away with eating the rice alone, you'll be in trouble. Protein from the chicken would have seeped into every little grain and will have rendered it a miscombination.

- To ensure the highest quality of energy when eating open-with-discretion meals, stay in the same family of foods: fish with other fish or shellfish, eggs with chicken, two kinds of pasta. Different kinds of food generate different kinds of energy. But please don't just take my word for it; experience it for yourself and experience the "new you."

D A Y   3 0

Prunes
Vegetable Sandwich
Vegetable Ethnic/Open Carbohydrate

Even though your Skinny future is going to include as many miscombination meals as you can get away with, you might choose for the most part to play it straight. I know I do. Why? Well, for one thing, I usually eat too much when I miscombine and suffer the consequences—added weight. But more important, I don't feel as well when I miscombine as when I stick to the categories. Believe me, if you use your imagination, "straight" meals don't have to be boring. See the examples in "Playing It Straight" (p. 115), for a few ideas to get you started.

Although tonight's meal is going to be all carbohydrates, you're not locked in to just plain, steamed vegetables. Why not go ethnic . . . Indian, Chinese, Middle Eastern, even Mexican (but watch the cheese)?

Now it's time for you to start doing your own scheduling. This is something you'll have to learn how to do if you want eternal slimhood to be a reality because even when you've achieved your goal you are still going to have to think about food and plan what you are going to eat. Don't worry, it's easy to do once you know how.

Once you have achieved your goal, you'll no longer think about your weight on a daily basis, but rather on a weekly basis. You'll continue to weigh yourself daily, as I said before, but no one can be so firm that their weight will not fluctuate from day to day, but it should never fluctuate by more than three pounds and it should remain constant from one week to the next.

Since you probably know your business and social schedule a week in advance, it's best to build your program around what you have planned. Remember, if you plan for it, if you schedule it in, nothing is fattening. And remember, don't deprive or be stingy with yourself.

Take a piece of paper and divide it into the seven days of the week. Schedule in all business and social commitments first, then your emotional ones. Think of what you want to eat and when you want to eat it. Mark your choices on your weekly chart first, then fill in the blanks. What you choose to eat will determine what you have to eat the rest of the week. For instance, if I know in advance that Thursday lunch I'm going to eat pizza, then the first blank I'll fill in is my breakfast for that day. I'll check the precedote list in "Corrective Counterparts" (p. 111) to see what I should eat before greasy, creamy, cheesy foods: it's pineapple. Then, I'll fill in my dinner. The pizza has protein in it, so that dictates that I must eat 80 percent protein for dinner. And so it goes day to day. Now tally up your nutritional quotient for the week (60 percent carbs, 20 percent to 25 percent protein, 20 percent fats), making sure that you have the proper amount of protein, carbs and fats. Be sure that you are feeding your body the nutrients it needs. And do not, I repeat, do not slight your emotional needs. Remember, *The New Beverly Hills Diet* program is for every aspect of you, an individualized program that must cater to your heart if it is to be "forever."

When we started together, I told you I would never take your heart out of your stomach. I was just going to put your head in. I was going to make you think a little. *The New Beverly Hills Diet* program means *thinking* about food. But unlike your food thoughts of the past, instead of the "should's" and "should not's," the "can't's" and "never's," instead of your food consciousness being ruled by ignorance, apathy, myths and your fat consciousness, it's going to be propelled by knowledge, understanding, positive food thoughts and choices.

You have a choice now, a choice that is no longer to eat or not to eat, but what to eat and when to eat it in order to make it work best.

Soon, I'm no longer going to be responsible for telling you what to eat. I'm relinquishing that decision to you. You'll take my hints and my suggestions, but you'll make your own decisions, decisions that will be dictated by later and tomorrow instead of right now, instead of just today. This is your diet, your eating plan, and to make it work it must be based on your food and your choices.

I know I've said it over and over, but weigh yourself every day and write it down. Never compromise your love affair with your scale, which is your impartial judge of Skinny. Don't be afraid of it.

Again, you absolutely must schedule your weeks in advance. Resist that temptation to "wing it." Resist the temptation to leave them open, to be spontaneous "to see what happens." You know what will happen . . . and you'll only be sorry.

When you begin scheduling, always plan for the possibility of added pounds. Prepare for the worst by always scheduling in the maximum corrective counterparts. As you develop your maintenance profile, as you begin to see what your body can handle, you'll be able to ease up a little. As you learn what your body will tolerate, and as your body learns to respond to *The New Beverly Hills Diet* program, Conscious Combining will become automatic and you'll move into the world of "Unconscious Combining." I know by experience that I can get away with eating four and a half pieces of pizza in a single night and not gain an ounce. I also know that if I eat four and a half pieces of pizza the next night, I will inevitably put on one and a half pounds. I've experimented with this time and time again. I know my weight gain score for all my favorite foods and even my not-so-favorite foods. Right now you only need to experiment with and experience your favorites. Why bother with the others? Remember, I had to experiment because I was creating a universal methodology, an eating program that would include all of you.

I haven't suggested anything to you that my clients and I haven't experienced ourselves. Always remember that *The New Beverly Hills Diet* program is experiential as well as theoretical. We Conscious Combiners know what works and what doesn't because we've tried it all.

DAY 31

Orange Juice and Choice of Cantaloupe, Honeydew or Half a Grapefruit
Sandwich of Choice
Protein

Just in case you've missed your former "diet" breakfast, I thought I'd give you a reminder of what you once thought you'd have to do to stay thin. This morning you're going to have juice and melon. Eat it, finish it and then you're through until lunch and no picking in between. Not so easy, is it?

Lunch, however, is a different story. You're on *The New Beverly Hills Diet* Born-Again Skinny program, so go for it! Have the sandwich of your choice with all the trimmings. Think about it, though. Knowing what you now know, does it really have to be a chili cheese dog? How about an all-vegetarian sandwich, like avocado? Remember, what you choose to eat determines what you have to eat. So if you choose a miscombination sandwich, that would dictate an 80-percent-protein dinner. Exactly what do I mean by 80 percent? It means that if you can't live without bread and butter before a meal, have some (but then, that's your carb). If prime rib isn't prime rib without a baked potato, add one to your plate, but stop there.

I repeat: Every miscombination does not a fat person make, not if you engage in that miscombination with discretion and without adding insult to injury. You know what I mean . . . as long as you have dropped the attitude of, "Well, since I've had bread I might as well have a salad, oh heck, sure, bring me the baked potato . . ." *Only you can make miscombinations work.* So miscombine with that thought in mind. When you can make miscombinations work for you, you can have them all the time.

Just how many "open meals" you'll be able to get away with in a day, a week and a month will depend entirely on you. Experience and experimentation will give you the answer, and only time will tell.

Remember, when you're eating an open meal, you'll have to exercise more discipline. You'll have to enlist the aid of your Skinny voice and listen closely for it to proclaim, "Enough already!" Your stomach probably won't be hearing anything, not if the food still tastes good. The pizza at Due's in Chicago tastes good to me until I literally can't fit any more in. If I ask for and finish the extra fries every time I have my "cheeseburger from paradise" at Duke's in Seattle, or go hog wild every time I have barbecue at Mississippi Flyway in Carbondale, my Skinny little wings will be clipped and I'm going to chunk on the pounds, and it's not worth it. Overindulging means paying the price, pruning your pleasure and triggering the pain of guilt.

Test, taste and try. Know your limits because only you can set them. Put your mind into your eating and evoke your good common sense.

At the end of two or three months, you should have a fairly firm fix on just how much you can get away with and just how far you can go. Test your limits and, as the weeks go by, increase your pleasures and gradually increase your miscombinations. Now, when I say increase, I'm not suggesting that each week you double your pleasure. Add one miscombination at a time. Be gentle and ease into it. Monitor your progress each step along the way, reveling in what you can get away with and drawing the line where you must. You'll find that it's a mighty skinny line that marks the difference between thin and fat.

Something as innocuous as added salt, a diet drink, a mediocre sauce or a handful of nuts at the wrong time can spell gained pounds.

Experience, experiment and enjoy. But, I repeat, *ease* into it. Trust in *The New Beverly Hills Diet* program. You know it works! Your new body and way of thinking prove it. Each *New Beverly Hills Diet* Skinny maintainer is testimony to the power of the enzyme, and you will be, too.

Initially, because of your fat potential and past history your body probably won't tolerate too many miscombinations. Don't panic because the miscombinations probably won't make your body feel very well. Stay aware of how you feel because it is every bit as important to maintaining as what your scale tells you. After all, feeling terrific is the bottom line; everything else relates to that—your weight, your emotions and your new *thin* world.

DAY 32

Protein

When you're on an all-protein day like today, you should plan on trying to make it a three-meal-only day. Eat until you're full at each meal, and when you're done, you're done. Keep nibbling to a minimum. There are several reasons for restricting between-meal eating on all-protein days. Physically, you'll confuse the enzymes. How? When you eat protein, you first excrete hydrochloric acid from your stomach walls to burn up the fat. Once that fat has been taken care of, the hydrochloric acid shuts off and pepsin comes along to do its "softening" job (remember the bam bam bam of the hammer). When pepsin has completed its initial task, it is joined by hydrochloric acid to complete the breakdown of protein into amino acids. This three-step process begins anew each time a new protein enters the stomach. If a new protein is added while Step 3 is going on, that action has to stop so that the newer protein can be accommodated with Step 1.

The one thing we don't ever want to stop is any action, including that hand-to-mouth action, except on all-protein days. Not snacking today should be easy because all-protein days are days when you can really appreciate being full . . . not stuffed, not bloated, just not wanting or needing to eat. All-protein days (particularly meat protein) can be quite effective in conquering excess water retention. The meat acts like a mop sopping up the extra water. You'll notice that it appears with watermelon on your antidote list in "Corrective Counterparts" (p. 111). Meat works like a charm when used in moderation— never more than one all-protein day per week. This does not, however, exclude individual protein meals at other times during the week.

Speaking of working, have you been wondering if your scale has stopped working? Has it been stuck on one place for a while? Or perhaps, this already happened to you and you've gotten beyond it. If it hasn't, look out because it's inevitable. It's called a plateau, one of those inevitable unannounced places we all reach when the weight loss stops. Day after day, we get on the scale, and no matter how good we've been, we don't get our reward; the scale doesn't budge. How did we deal with this in the past? By eating, of course. Out of frustration, we'd shove the food in. If you can't lose, you may as well gain, right? At least the scale moves—even if it's the wrong way.

Plateaus can be easy to bear if you understand a little bit about what they really are.

On a purely physical level, the fat has to get out of your body. It has to be softened and burned before it is ultimately flushed out and eliminated. This doesn't happen in an instant. First, fat leaves the cells and travels to the appropriate channel of elimination (kidneys and large intestine) before exiting your body.

What remains are the cells where the fat resided— and they don't just disappear. After the fat is gone the cells fill with water. They came into being because there was extra food to be had. Now they aren't leaving, they're waiting to be fed again. Eventually, the cells get the message that you're not going to feed them. Speck by speck, they begin to shrink, and so do you.

If you become conscious of this process (by doing your mirror exercise), you'll realize that while the scale isn't so much as flickering, your body is changing quite dramatically. Hang in there. The water that is gradually leaving the cell will ultimately be flushed out. You never know when a plateau will strike or just how long it will last.

During my final weight loss, when I was "going all the way," I got stuck for a full 13 days at 112 pounds despite desperate measures. Once I had proved to myself that I wouldn't give in to fat, once I had proved that I would not succumb to the lure of cashews or raisins or anything else I wanted to eat, I began losing again. The following week, eight pounds dropped off.

Plateaus are not only physical, they are emotional as well. In fact, they are emotional more often than not.

Plateaus give us time to catch up to our new bodies. They allow our heads and bodies time to get back in sync. If you have lost, say, 12 pounds, you're experiencing life from an entirely different vantage point. You don't have the 12 pounds of padding and armor that you once had. You're more vulnerable and you need to consciously assimilate your new being. Take advantage of the plateau to do just that. In reality, you're a different entity every time you lose a single pound.

For years, we've either been on a diet trying to lose weight or we've been off our diet, which means we're gaining. Do you ever remember just being—neither losing nor gaining? Have you ever simply stopped and said, "This is where I am right now"? So often we are so obsessed with our final goal, which may be some 10 or 30 pounds away, that we don't stop to experience now, to feel today. Plateaus are breathing spaces. If you let them be, plateaus can be highly positive. Experience yourself where you are **now.** Not where you've been, not where you're going. . . . **Now!**

Plateaus give you an opportunity to make a choice. You can always eat; that's probably what you have done in the past, and it is one of the reasons you've never been able to get thin. All the frustrations, the anxieties, the hostilities and the depressions you feel each day as you weigh yourself are only feelings you've had before. Feel them and let them go. You don't have to swallow them anymore. You know the scale will eventually move again . . . that it will keep going down.

By this time you have probably lost about 15 pounds. That's equal to about seven chickens. (A chicken weighs about two pounds.) Do you feel it? Are you looking at yourself naked in the mirror? Have you been doing your daily dance or walk in place?

Outlasting a plateau means stating your case and saying, "This is forever. I will do whatever it takes. I want to be thin more than anything, even food." Once you're willing to give up anything, there's only one thing you'll have to give up, and that's your fat.

Before you can choose not to be fat, you have to understand what makes you fat. Only then can you rid yourself of it and become thin.

Plateaus make you confront that fat person and they force your hand. This is the test. Are you really committed? Are you willing to go the distance? Do you have what it takes to be Skinny? *The New Beverly Hills Diet* program and Conscious Combining give you all the tools you'll ever need. Use them!

You do have what it takes, you know. You have proved it by coming this far. So just give it up and let it go—your fat, that is. WELCOME, SLIMHOOD!

P.S. If you're in a quandary about what to eat today, you will find perfectly combined protein meals in "Playing It Straight" (p. 115).

DAY 33

Pineapple
Two Bananas

Day 33 and you're almost home free.

Okay, Skinny, we're going out with a bang—or should I say a bam bam. These next two days should give any leftover fat quite a jolt, and then we'll use our trusty watermelon to wash it all out.

I'm wondering, have you been keeping up with your what-you-love-about-being-thin and hate-about-fat lists? Today or, better yet, tonight before you go to bed, pull them out and make some additions, particularly on the what-I-hate-about-being-fat page. Fat is a thing of the past, so let's bury it! I don't want you to think about being fat anymore. When you close your eyes tonight there's just one thing I want you to think about: How great it is to be thin!

What is *so great about being thin?* It means going to bed feeling good about yourself. (Does anything make you feel worse than being fat?) For so many years we've been absorbed by our bodies—with being thin, with how we feel, and especially with how we look. Somehow we've been victimized into believing we have no responsibility, no choice.

We either have a slow metabolism or an under active thyroid, it's genetic, our parents were fat, we're doomed to be fat because we love to eat, and loving to eat and being thin are mutually exclusive.

We've become so sophisticated about food, and its meaning has become so convoluted in our minds, that we've mentally smothered its simple and original purpose. It creates our flesh and blood, and is our energy. Food will always be an excuse for a social situation, an emotional stopgap, an expression of love, an instant and temporary cure for boredom. Eating will always be a time for families to get together, to celebrate, to rejoice and unite. It's a time to do business, it's a reward and it's a punishment. These are all true, but above all, food is you. You are what you eat—pure and simple—no more, no less.

Our lives, our food, our eating have been dictated by habit and tradition. Our hearts, rather than our heads, have ruled our eating. As I'm sure you realize by now, I'm the last person to take your heart out of your stomach. I know how it feels. I have those moments of madness when my head says no but my heart says go, and most of the time, I listen to my heart. That's okay because my choice in those moments of madness doesn't have to be *not* to eat, but rather *what* to eat to make it work. What to eat to stay thin and feel good.

As an "eater," you know that those moments of madness happen quite frequently. What has saved me, what has kept me skinny, and what will save you and keep you skinny, is strict adherence to the four Golden Rules. These rules are as important to me as the moral code that guides my life. Just as I wouldn't commit murder, I wouldn't break these rules, either. The Golden Rules have the potential to ensure your eternal slimhood.

The other rules and tools I have told you about, while all vitally important, can be broken occasionally without fat taking over or your energy being instantly zapped. But no matter how flagrantly I may abuse any of the other rules, never do I trifle with the Golden Rules. The Golden Rules are sacred, never to be abused.

Keep in mind that the rules and tools were first discovered when I was seeking my personal cure for fat, when I was struggling alone through that mire of misery. There were a few physical laws to guide me, but the methodology, the philosophy, the rules and the tools all came first out of my own personal experience and experiments, and later out of those of my clients. People often ask me, "Didn't you break the rules when you first started, didn't you slip up once in a while?" I remind them that there were no "rules" when I started, I had to make them up. The rules as we know them are simply a product of what did and didn't work. They only became etched in stone as they were stretched to their limits, as I went along and experimented.

Since then, with the help of well over a thousand Beverly Hills Dieters whom I personally supervised in my Beverly Hills clinic and later all over the world, I've experimented and refined, honed and hacked. Only then did I put the "Golden Rules" down indelibly as guidelines for all of us (p. 104). Believe me, my clients and I have tried stretching them to the limit. We know that the Golden Rules cannot—must not—be violated.

Again, I'm asking you to take these rules and put them on a pedestal, to internalize them so that they always guide your eating, to make them as much a part of your life, as much a part of your moral code, as I have done. Establish these few simple guidelines when it comes to eating. Make that commitment to me and to yourself. Remember, you're not eliminating anything from your life, you're adding to it, and together we will revel in the power of the hipbones and frolic in the land of forever skinny!

DAY 34

Pineapple
Papaya
Pineapple

If you think about food when it doesn't count, you won't have to think about it when it does.

Try making your home a Conscious Combiner's haven. Promise yourself that your home will be a sanctuary for feeling good and staying skinny. It's easy. Stock your shelves, fridge and freezer. Get rid of the packaged goods that are loaded with preservatives and chemicals; give them away, or better yet throw them out. Learn to adapt your favorite recipes and try some wonderful new ones. Remember, make every bite count. Why would you even have commercially processed oil in your house once you've started using cold-pressed, or for that matter, lite mayonnaise made with fat substitutes, TV dinners, crackers with lard and sodium propionate, peanut butter with salt and hydrogenated oil, salty potato chips or sugary breakfast cereals?

Remember, there is a healthy equivalent for even the most unhealthy food. Your home should house only the best, and the rules and the tools should be the gospel. It's your choice, your territory. The more good you do when you can, the more bad you can do when you want or have to.

The first giant step I took toward slimhood and health was eliminating foods with preservatives and chemicals from my kitchen. I prided myself on having what I called an "organic" home. As I explained earlier, the human body was not created to process all those artificial ingredients and it has to figure out what, if anything, it can do with them. Many of them don't get processed at all. They just stay stored in the body. Others, during processing, cause damage to our bodies' vitamin and mineral supplies as well as impede the digestive process. Save the junk for the outside, where you don't have any quality control. You'll be able to feed your heart and soul when you want to, if you feed your body when you can.

Now, moving on to a few specifics:

- If you haven't already tossed out your salt shaker, do it now. There really is no excuse for eating salt at home. Remember, whether you're a "bloater" or not, your body can only handle so much salt without retaliating. Save salt for the outside, for when you have no choice, or for those foods that don't exist without it.
- Use unsalted butter.
- Always have enough of *The New Beverly Hills Diet* foods in reserve. Don't set yourself up for failure by running out of core foods. There should be a hefty supply of pineapple and papaya ripening on your window sill and lying in wait in your refrigerator, as

well as dried fruits such as prunes, raisins and apricots, plus a supply of raw nuts and seeds safely stowed away.

- Stop buying canned vegetables. Most contain salt and chemicals. Frozen vegetables, however, are handy to have around and will do in a pinch.
- Share *The New Beverly Hills Diet* with your family. Cook them Consciously Combined meals and they will not only love them, they will feel fabulous and will probably be more fun to live with.
- Save your open meals for when you go out. While at home, play it straight. Why stretch it when you don't have to, when it probably won't be for anything too terrific anyhow? When you realize the straight splendors you can create in your own kitchen, your chubby little soul will be in perpetual ecstasy. Besides which, at home you can make and have as much of anything as you want.
- Clean out those closets. Throw out your fat clothes. Go shopping. Get a new hairdresser or barber and get a new haircut.
- Fill your house with mirrors. Reinforce your emotional high by looking at your body and rejoicing in its perfection.

DAY 35

Watermelon or Grapes

The good life is yours—welcome to forever!

You did it, you found that pot of gold at the end of the rainbow: Eternal slimhood. You've earned it, so be proud of yourself because I'm proud of you. You have entered the good life, the land of plenty: plenty of food, plenty of fun and plenty of time to enjoy it. You have created a life for yourself that is a dream come true. And now you know for sure, now you really believe that you can be as thin as you'd like for the rest of your life without giving up anything, without ever being deprived. You know this because you've done it. You're experiencing the wonders of the good life, a life that includes everything you have ever wanted. Food is now your slave and you are the master; it works for you, not against you.

All the shame and degradation, the heartache and hunger, the diet and deprivation are banished. They no longer exist. They are gone forever. You've smashed that miserable, debilitating fat cycle, you erased the tape. Your fat consciousness has been pushed aside by your Skinny voice. You're not fat anymore and you'll never be fat again.

Five weeks ago I told you there were three things you were going to have to give up if you wanted skinny to become a forever reality. As you gave up your fat, as you gave up your guilt, and as, one by one, you let go of all your preconceived ideas about fat and fattening, diets and dieting, you replaced them with a pride and self-confidence you never knew you possessed. You've taken control of the essence of your life and put it to work for you. You have learned to exploit the synergy of your mind and body. You are powerful. Your hipbones and cheekbones are the joyful testimony to your success.

You have spent the last five weeks understanding, accepting and internalizing the concept of tomorrow, the concept of forever that will keep you thin. That is the heart of *The New Beverly Hills Diet* program. A tomorrow that only existed in your wildest fantasies is here, a tomorrow that is now a reality, a tomorrow free from fear.

Well, tomorrow is here for you to celebrate. Could you have imagined getting on your scale and not having to lose one more pound? Could you have imagined being perfect? Did you ever realize how much of your life was colored by fat?

Did you ever imagine a tomorrow that includes everything you ever wanted to eat; a tomorrow that allows you to eat to your heart's content without eating your heart out? Did you ever imagine a tomorrow where you would be totally in control; where the old diet consciousness would be banished forever? Did you ever think you'd be able to make food work for you, not by giving it up but just by unlocking its enzymes?

At long last, you can have your cake and eat it, too. Does it really matter if you have to eat it one piece at a time? One by one, all your excuses have been stripped away. There's nothing out there you can't eat. Nothing. You've eliminated your greatest obstacle to slimhood . . . you.

Gone forever is the fat consciousness, the wallowing in self-pity, the obsession with negatives. Gone forever is the desperation, the desolation, the resignation and the guilt of being fat forever. No longer does skinny mean hunger, deprivation and a black cloud of "never's." No longer will food sap your power and energy. You have learned how to manipulate food, how to use it to maximize your energy, how to use it to keep you thin.

Here forever is a reality that includes everything you ever wanted. Here forever is a diet that is a way of life, a dream come true, a diet where nothing is fattening; a diet that builds in antidotes for blowing it; in which, no matter what you eat, there are corrective counterparts to erase its effects; a diet that feeds your body instead of starving it.

For the first time in your life you have permission to enjoy food, to make food an experience and to experience food. For the first time in your life, you have embraced a way of eating that is built around the foods you love. What you choose to eat determines what you have to eat. You never have to cheat to get what you want because there's no diet to break. This is your diet, not somebody else's, and it's forever.

You don't have to prove anything anymore. You have made a commitment. You have put your mind and your intellect into eating. You have learned to make conscious choices. You have shed the fat-perpetuating diet consciousness forever.

For the first time in your life you have glorious energy, a body you can be proud of, and the ammunition to keep it that way for the rest of your life.

You've never looked or felt better, your hair gleams, your eyes glisten, your skin radiates. You wake up invigorated, you need less sleep, and best of all you feel great about yourself. You are all that you hoped you could be. You have grasped the core of the good life and all it has to offer.

You have learned to listen and respond to your body. You experience food, and you understand that how it makes you feel is far more important than how it tastes. Because you now understand the totality of food you realize that you are a product of what you eat, nothing more, nothing less. You have learned to love the foods that make you feel good and to love the foods that merely taste good a little less. Your heart understands and agrees.

Eating is no longer just a function of your emotions, a reaction, a habit. It is now a pleasure. It is nourishment. It is a positive. In becoming a thin person, you confronted, acknowledged and let go of the fat person. You discarded your cloak of secrecy; now everyone knows who you are and what you are. They know that you're an "eater" and you aren't ashamed of it. Well, why should you be? You're no longer wearing the negative side effects! You don't have to pretend to be someone you're not, you don't have to conjure up excuses, you can openly enjoy eating, you can unleash your wildest fantasies and fetishes. When you detail the raptures of a mango, bask in the delights of a meal eaten yesterday, or eagerly anticipate an eating experience three days away, you don't worry. You don't care what other people think. You have permission to experience food and make it an experience. You have all the security and power of a thin person, a person no longer ashamed of who you are.

With your new food security blanket, you can have whatever you want, whenever you want. You can eat a chocolate soufflé for lunch, you can have popcorn for breakfast, or sunny-side up eggs for dinner. When it comes to food, you can have it your way.

You are experiencing how food energizes your body instead of draining it. You have pioneered the ultimate transformation. Instead of eating to bring yourself down, as a refuge from misery, you eat for the pluses: the pleasure and the power. For the first time in your life you are satisfied, you'll never be hungry again—not for food, not for anything. You have achieved the most difficult goal in your life and now that you've done that, now that you're skinny, you can do and have anything. Your Skinny person is in control and you are all-powerful.

Your scale has indeed become your best friend, it has become an integral part of your life, it is your point of reference, your foundation of reality. Your weight is no longer your measure of good and bad, but rather a guidepost to what does and doesn't work. It is a barometer that tallies your state of being, not a noose around your conscience. Every time you get on that scale and celebrate not having to lose one more pound, each time you leap on that scale and experience the high of saying, "I'm perfect," you've cemented one more Skinny block in place and you can put fat that much farther behind you. Now that you can luxuriate in your perfect weight, you can let your fantasies run free. Now you have summoned forever!

If you can maintain for six months, you can be skinny forever. The first months of maintenance are the scourge of the golden pineapple, the nemesis of the good life, mentally, emotionally and physically. They really put you to the test. It is during the first treacherous six months, as the cleansing process continues, while your body is stabilizing in spurts and sputters and your brain is absorbing, assimilating and adjusting, that you are moving from the negative to the positive; that you are discarding your fat consciousness and replacing it with skinny. You are fixing the golden pineapple forever in your heart.

While each week that passes reinforces skinny and undermines fat, never forget from whence you came. Fat and lethargy are as near as tomorrow. They will stop at nothing to reclaim you. Nothing. Now that you have embraced the good life, hold on. Don't give in and don't ever give up. Don't dwell on your fat consciousness; you did that long enough. Just know that it's there, poised to prey on your vulnerabilities. Revel in the forever of skinny, hold on tight, and don't let go. Rejoice in it, appreciate it and enjoy it. You've earned it.

You know, I need your success, too. You're my reason for doing all this. Your success is my success. You are the living, breathing proof that there is a cure for fat, and that skinny isn't a transient phenomenon.

Conscious Combining means eternal slimhood. You've helped change the statistics. Let me welcome you into the world of forever.

Although you are now on your own, I'm not worried. I know you can do it. You have become part of a very special network of Skinnies, and we will be linked together always.

. . . Now you have it all: hamburgers and hipbones, cheesecake and cheekbones. You are indeed a Conscious Combiner of the first order.

Congratulations, Skinny, I'm proud of you.

Born-Again Skinny
Phase Two

Still have a way to go? Don't worry, I'm not going anywhere. I'm still here, I'm still with you. I'll be here for as long as it takes you.

Are you seeing yourself as the new you? The new Skinny you are on the way to becoming. A bridge isn't built before someone designs it. A skyscraper can't be erected before there is a blueprint. It all begins with an idea—an image. And that includes your new body.

I know it's tough; you've grown accustomed to that old fat image and a mere loss of pounds won't necessarily change that, not if you're still wearing those same old clothes, still sporting that same old haircut—the 'do that went with the old you.

So on this watermelon day, let's not just wash out that fat; let's also wash out that old fat image. Buy yourself a new outfit, get yourself a new haircut and then look in the mirror and see the new you!

Okay, so you aren't perfect yet. You haven't achieved your goal. Well, it's only a matter of time. Meanwhile, just continue doing what you've been doing—eating, enjoying and getting thinner. Come on, these past 35 days haven't exactly been torture. True, not every day has been hamburgers from heaven, but then how many days were "heaven" when you were fat? How much of your old eating did you really enjoy (beyond, of course, those few moments the food was in your mouth)? You don't want to go back to that, do you? Of course not. And there are several ways to continue.

We've already talked at length about maintenance; now let's spend some time discussing how you'll continue losing weight. These past 35 days will provide you with a strong foundation.

Continued weight loss is a cinch, so just cinch that belt one notch tighter and let's go for it. How? Well, you could go back to Day 1 and start all over again. But don't. The surprise is gone. It's too repetitious and you'll get bored. Instead, pick up at any day—the day won't matter. What does matter is your commitment to follow it through in seven-day increments. The days are in a carefully planned sequence, each juxtaposed to the next specifically for nutritional and enzymatic reasons. The important thing is that you do seven days in a row. Trust me, if you don't, it won't work. Now, of course, you can do more than seven days in a row, but the minimum when taking the diet out of context is seven. If you didn't fare so well on your last open days, go back to your diet diary and your rehash sheets. What did you eat and what are you now willing to eliminate? Go a little easier, eat some new things, things you didn't have the last time. It won't be as hard this time now that you truly understand that *nothing is leaving the planet.*

Take a week off now and then, and go on a maintenance week. Schedule it the way I described on Day 30.

Each time you start a new week, reread that section. Let me help you, let me help strengthen your
Skinny aura. You'll lose, you'll get thin. Maybe it
won't be tomorrow, but each tomorrow will bring you
closer and closer to the dream that is soon to become
a reality. So don't give up, just give in; give in to thin.
Soon that tomorrow of forever will be here for you, too.

Notes

_____

_____

_____

_____

_____

_____

_____

_____

_____

_____

_____

_____

Notes *(continued)*

CONGRATULATIONS!

Your victory is living testimony to the wonders of *The New Beverly Hills Diet* program. Your success shouts it out. Your glow breathes life into Conscious Combining, giving hope to millions of fatties who are waiting to see, waiting to hear—those who needed more proof, those less eager than you to be on the cutting edge.

We've not only discovered how we can be as thin as we'd like for the rest of our lives, we've done it. If we can do it, so can others. Take up the challenge and join me in Pineappleland, where we can shout our victory.

Once you have completed your initial 35 days, mail me a copy of your diet diary and your before and after pictures, as well as some comments about your experiences. Add a self-addressed, stamped envelope and I'll send you a graduation certificate—or should I say a birth certificate for a *Born-Again Skinny*. Send these glowing reports to:

Judy Mazel
ClubSlim
Inn at Queen Anne
505 First Avenue North
Seattle, WA 98109
800-999-6129
(206) 283-4508

You're also invited to join me and other Skinnies on the World Wide Web for chats, support and sharing at *The New Beverly Hills Diet* homepage:

http://www.cyberskinny.com